DO-IT-YOURSELF
HERBAL
MEDICINE

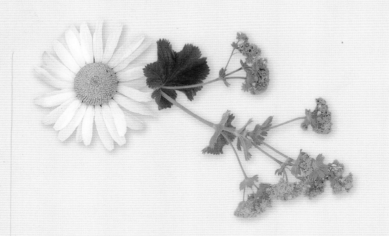

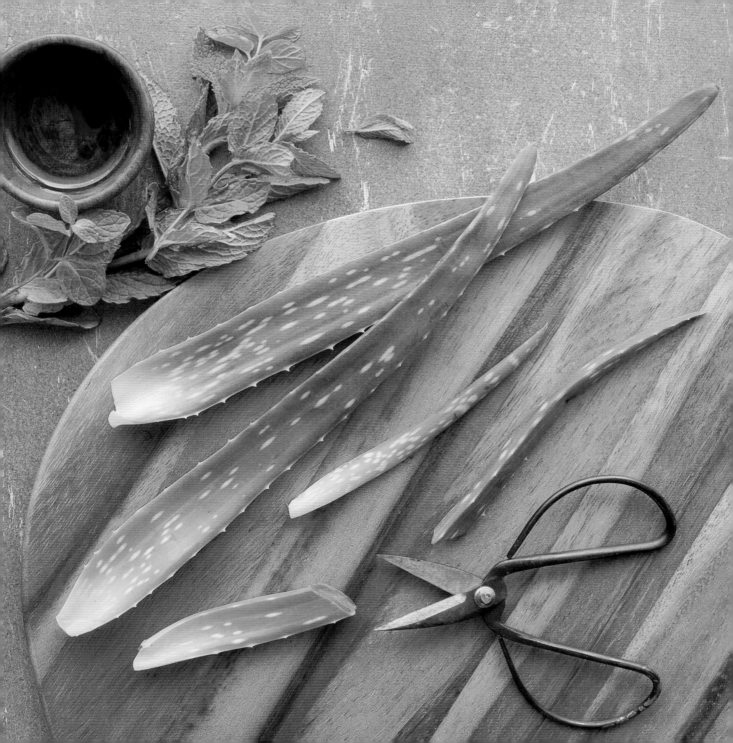

Home-Crafted Remedies
for Health & Beauty

DO-IT-YOURSELF
HERBAL
MEDICINE

FALL RIVER PRESS

New York

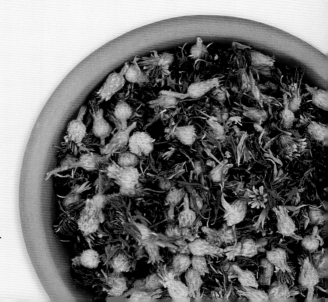

FALL RIVER PRESS

New York

An Imprint of Sterling Publishing Co., Inc.
1166 Avenue of the Americas
New York, NY 10036

ISBN 978-1-4351-6286-0

For information about custom editions, special sales, and premium and corporate purchases,
please contact Sterling Special Sales at 800-805-5489 or specialsales@sterlingpublishing.com.

Manufactured in China

2 4 6 8 10 9 7 5 3

www.sterlingpublishing.com

Cover design by David Ter-Avanesyan

Photo credits: Shannon Oslick, pg. 1; Shannon Oslick, pg. 2; Shannon Oslick, pg. 6; Shannon Oslick, pg. 8;
Shannon Oslick, pg. 10-11; Shannon Oslick, pg. 12; s_bukley/shutterstock.com, pg. 22; Shannon Oslick, pg. 24;
Trinette Reed/Stocksy, pg. 30; Aleksandra Jankovic/Stocksy, pg. 31; Trinette Reed/Stocksy, pg. 33;
Carine Lutt/Stockfood, pg. 38; Foodcollection/Stockfood, pg. 39; Trinette Reed/Stocksy, pg. 40;
Trinette Reed/Stocksy, pg. 42; Bernard Radvaner/Media Bakery, pg. 43; Helga Esteb/Shutterstock.com,
pg. 44; Shannon Oslick, pg. 48-49; Shannon Oslick, pg. 50; Amy Convington/Stocksy, pg. 56; Shannon Oslick,
pg. 62; Shannon Oslick, pg. 94-95; Shannon Oslick, pg. 96; Laura Adani/Stocksy, pg. 107; Shannon Oslick,
pg. 122; Trinette Reed/Stocksy, pg. 133; Trinette Reed/Stocksy, pg. 147; Shannon Oslick, pg. 148; Sara
Remington/Stocksy, pg. 151; Shannon Oslick, pg. 164; Shannon Oslick, pg. 190; Kerry Murphy/Stocksy,
pg. 251; Shannon Oslick, pg. 252; Jill Chen/Stocksy, pg. 263; Shannon Oslick, pg. 274; Shannon Oslick, pg. 286.
All other photos iStock, Thinkstock, and Shutterstock.com.

CONTENTS

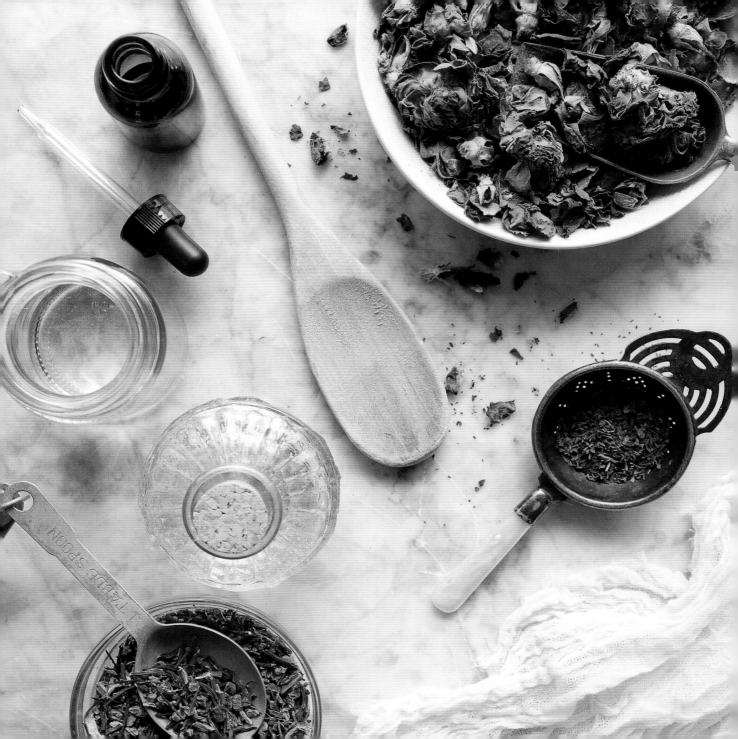

INTRODUCTION

You don't need to be a market researcher to know that herbal remedies are exploding in popularity. Do a quick search on Etsy. You'll see that crafters are doing more than knitting. The online emporium features skin care remedies, essential oils, soaps, sprays, salves, supplements, and more—all available for the curious herbal enthusiast. The wide range of products surely means that there is a market for herbal homemade alternatives.

So, who's using herbal medicine anyway?

Herbal medicine lingers on the periphery of the contemporary mindset much like an uninvited party guest (sure, we tolerate the *idea* of her, amusingly endure her antics, but she better not overstay her welcome). Yet more and more in the medical community, health-care providers and medical programs are incorporating natural remedies into their practices. There are even medical schools that combine conventional medicine with courses in herbal medicine and homeopathy—fusing standard science with alternative approaches in order to continually discover new ways to achieve balance in our bodies.

Yet despite herbal medicine's controversial status, more of us turn to it than you might think. According to the *New England Journal of Medicine*, nearly one-third of Americans use herbal medicine. But here's the thing: the same study found that 70 percent of people using herbal medicines are squeamish about acknowledging that to their doctor. Why the embarrassment? Why are so many of us seeking out

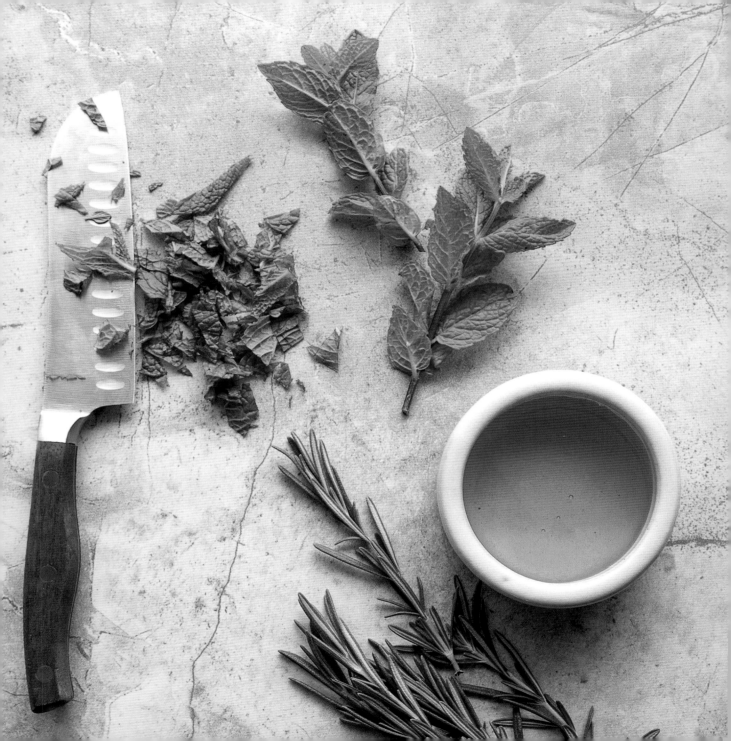

herbal remedies yet reluctant to admit to it? Maybe it's the taboo shroud, the prevailing sense that "complementary medicine" or "herbal remedies" are nothing more than modern buzzwords for witches' brew and old wives' tales. (*Rosehips? Garlic?* Sounds straight out of a Shakespearean drama, complete with cauldron emanating green smoke, right?)

But be honest. You've come to these pages because you have an interest in taking care of yourself naturally, and in reducing the amount of chemicals that make up your everyday routine—from your shampoo to the detergents you use to clean your home to the methods with which you treat common ailments. (By the way, that garlic in your pantry could come in handy to ward off infections, earaches, toothaches, and even pesky ants!

So, you're curious about herbal medicine. But you're not really sure where to start.

Maybe you swear by Method products. Maybe you want to guide your kids toward more mindful choices when it comes to their self-care. Or maybe you're choosing the homemade herbal route to save money.

Whatever your motivation, *Do-It-Yourself Herbal Medicine* provides the perfect starter guide for the DIY herbal novice. This comprehensive book will serve as a solid starting point as you learn more about the various herbs and their practical at-home uses. See Chapter 4 for the top thirty herbs to boost beauty and health. Then flip to Part 3: The Remedies to discover how to use these must-have herbs in everything from cosmetic concoctions to herbal healers to "day-after" remedies (to help you cope with the after-effects of a challenging breakup, late-night bar crawl, or wee-hours Netflix binge—we've all been there).

So whether you wish to make batches of body butter, or create chemical-free cleaners, or uncover DIY alternatives to boost your wellbeing, *Do-It-Yourself Herbal Medicine* will be your companion as you explore all that herbal medicine has to offer.

PART 1

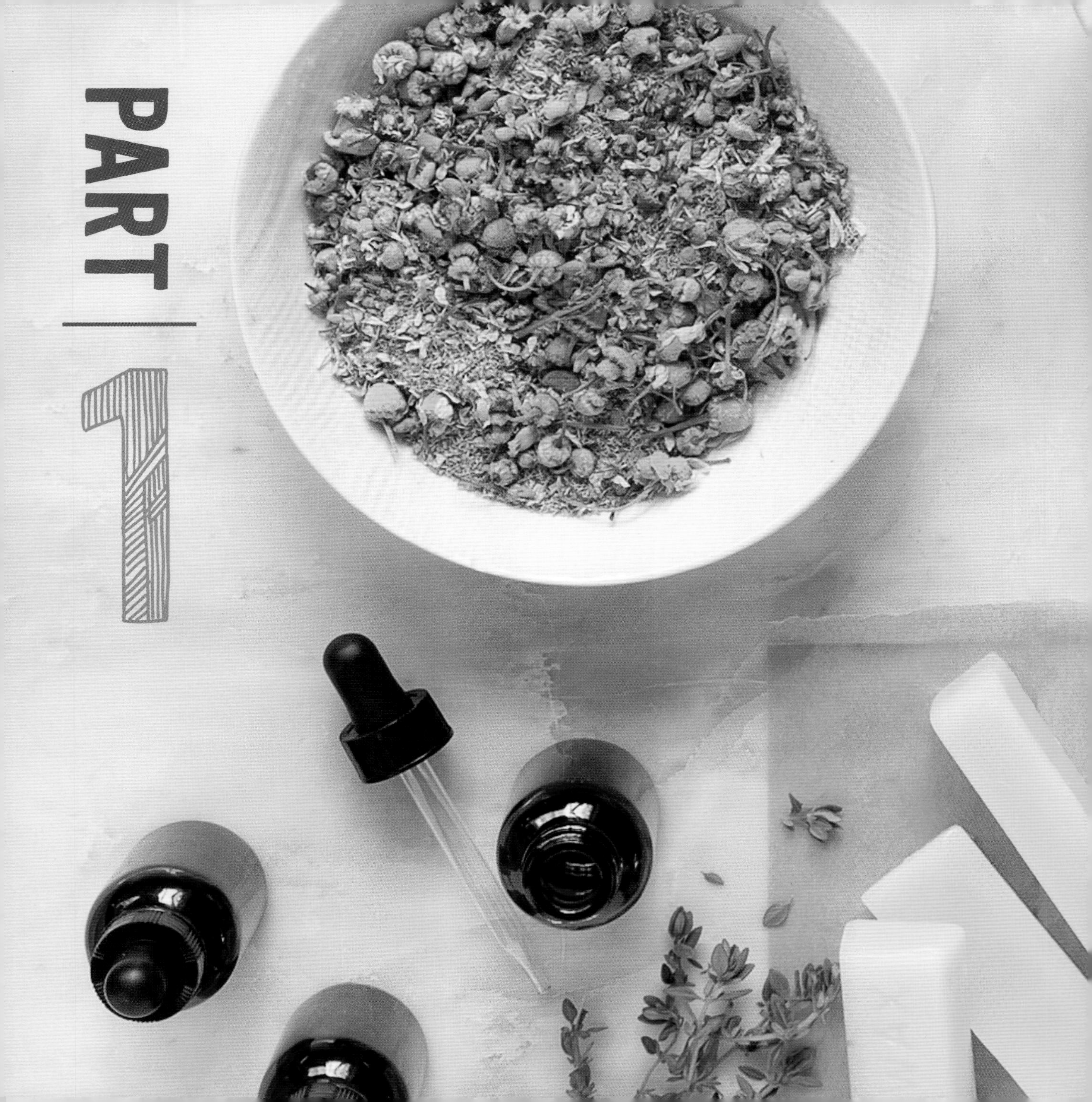

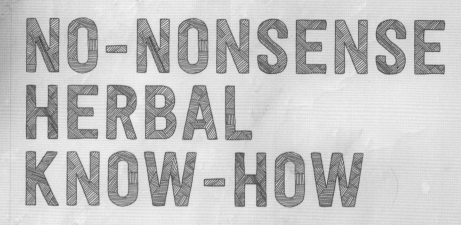

NO-NONSENSE HERBAL KNOW-HOW

Before you get your hands dirty, check out chapters 1 and 2 to find out all you need to know about the basics of DIY herbal medicine and how to make self-care fit into a modern lifestyle with optimal results. When finished, you'll be armed with must-have tools, easy tips, manageable shopping lists, and more. Have fun!

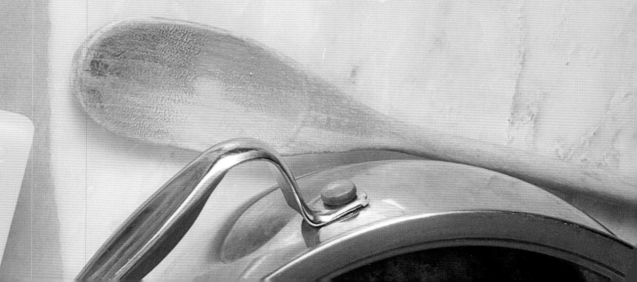

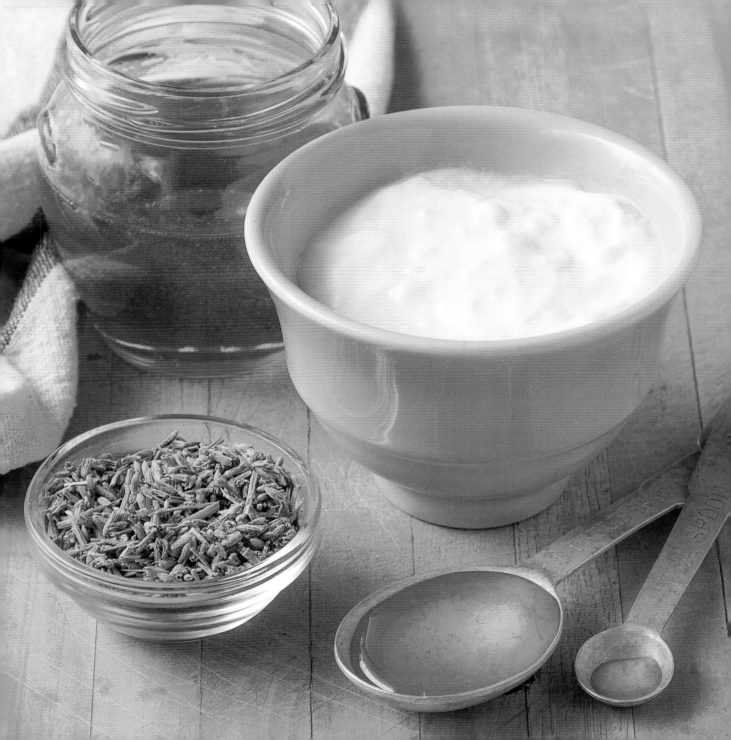

1

HERBAL MEDICINE AND YOU

A Modern Alternative

If you're like most people, herbal medicine is on your radar, but not necessarily in the most positive light. Maybe you envision herbal medicine as being for survivalists living off the grid, the Earth Mother hippie crowd boycotting "The System," or New Age healing circles shunning all things Western medicine. But even if it's nothing nearly so fringe that makes you roll your eyes—perhaps it's Gwyneth Paltrow's advocacy of herbal enemas?—there are still plenty of good reasons *not* to throw out the baby with the herbal bathwater.

Common issues we face every day—from acne, dry skin, or brittle hair to fatigue, mild depression, or stress—can be prevented, lessened, or treated through the targeted use of herb-infused lotions, shampoos, teas, and more. The good news is that you don't need to spend $18 on a scented candle from Anthropologie to satisfy your lavender fix or hunker down in the eucalyptus steam room at a luxury spa for aromatherapy benefits.

You may have heard that herbal medicine doesn't work, it's not rooted in science, or it's based on ancient principles that aren't relevant in a modern world. Truth is, there's a reason that herbs (and foods) have been used to heal, restore, and protect people from illness and injuries for centuries. Begin to understand this by exploring these common terms that are often tossed around like organic salad greens:

Essential oils are nutrient-dense volatile oils extracted from parts of a plant, like stems, leaves, flowers, and fruits, which give off a specific healing aroma.

Antioxidants are molecules found in plants, herbs, and food and they combat the harmful oxidizing agents that destroy cells. Antioxidants are necessary to repair or prevent cell damage and lessen your chance of disease.

Vitamins are substances your body gets from food in order to perform certain functions that it cannot perform on its own. Vitamins boost the immune system and are required for normal growth and development.

Essential oils, antioxidants, vitamins, and other healing compounds trigger our bodies to function efficiently, strengthen our immunity, and fight illness overall. Herbal preparations offer the vehicles for these healing agents to come into contact with our bodies. You're probably aware that many of these substances are extracted and studied by scientists, reengineered in labs, and made available in pharmaceutical prescriptions. By reading this book and dabbling with the recipes, you can get closer to the source of things—the piece of the equation that comes before prescriptions and reengineering.

In these pages, you'll get the straight talk about the most powerful healing herbs (without the brand pushes, company affiliations, or philosophical agendas), plus why they work and how to incorporate them into a modern household. Specifically, you'll get up to speed on the pros, cons, benefits, and suggested uses of a range of herbal preparations. By taking more of a complementary approach to health and beauty, it's likely your doctor's visits will start to be fewer and farther between.

WHAT IS HERBAL MEDICINE?

Put simply, *herbal medicine* involves the use of plants to prevent or treat illness. We know that the earliest civilizations used plant-based remedies. In fact, between 3,000 and 4,000 years ago humans recorded their use of many of the very same herbs we still use today for medicinal purposes. What might seem "New Age" to us in fact has deep historical roots.

Herbal Medicine Through the Ages—Briefly

Odds are you've heard of ginkgo biloba, even if you don't know much—or anything—about it. This plant contains antioxidants known as *flavonoids* that are used to improve cognitive functions. But did you know that scientists found fossilized specimens of ginkgo biloba dating to pre-dinosaur age (roughly 270 million years ago)? In Western herbalism, there are also documented records of ancient Egyptians using garlic to prevent and treat illness, as well as to enhance strength, and juniper oil for managing kidney and bladder diseases. These findings date back to 1700 BCE.

By 100 BCE the Greeks created a detailed methodology that connected different herbs to seasons, as well as to the elements of fire, air, earth, and water. In 77 CE, a Greek surgeon named Pedanius Dioscorides catalogued more than 600 plants and their uses in healing. The Romans later added to the Greek philosophies and a cataloguing system that is still used in medicine today. One example of this is the Roman concentration on prevention rather than cures.

Herbal treatments are also seen in early Eastern medicine traditions such as Traditional Chinese Medicine (TCM) and Ayurveda. The cultures of South America, Africa, Australia, and the South Pacific all have roots in herbal medicine. Australian aborigines, for example, discovered tea tree oil, a powerful antiseptic. Many healing herbs have been discovered in South American rainforests and mountains.

Ancient civilizations also used herbs for cosmetic purposes. In 1500 BCE, Egyptians documented the use of various herbs. Fenugreek, they noted, smoothed wrinkles; myrrh freshened the breath. Ancient Greeks used rose oils and waters to cleanse and hydrate skin. The same types of treatments are still quite popular today. You want shinier hair or a dandruff-free scalp? A nettle-based tonic will do the trick. No nettles? No problem. Parsley and rosemary work, too. Want more radiant, youthful-looking skin? Drink ginseng tea to brighten dullness, increase circulation, and combat dark circles.

ESSENTIAL OILS, ANTIOXIDANTS, VITAMINS, AND OTHER HEALING COMPOUNDS TRIGGER OUR BODIES TO FUNCTION EFFICIENTLY

TEST YOUR HERBAL IQ

Answer these 10 questions to check your smarts

1. ___ percent of the world's population uses herbal medicine.

A. 50   C. 20
B. 80   D. 5

2. The World Health Organization (WHO) estimates that ____ plant species are used around the world for medicinal purposes.

A. 3,000   C. 7,000
B. 5,000

3. Medicinal herbs come from which part of the plant:

A. stem   E. seeds
B. leaf   F. all of the
C. roots   above
D. bark

4. The global market for herbs and supplements will hit $ _____ by 2017.

A. 150 billion   C. 50 billion
B. 107 billion   D. 90 billion

5. True or False: Aromatherapy is based on scent alone.

6. The WHO reports that ___ percent of the drugs used in the United States are derived from plants.

A. 25   C. 75
B. 50   D. 10

7. ___ percent of medical schools offer alternative medicine courses or degrees.

A. 25   C. 75
B. 60   D. 33

8. ____ percent of Fortune 500 companies include alternative medicine in their health care plans.

A. 35   C. 70
B. 50   D. 19

9. The National Institutes of Health (NIH) invests $___ million annually in research on complementary and alternative medicine.

A. 10   C. 60
B. 40   D. 80

10. ___ percent of Americans use alternative or complementary medicine.

A. 25   C. 55
B. 40   D. 10

ANSWERS 1. B. 80 ■ 2. C. 7,000 ■ 3. F. all of the above ■ 4. B. 107 billion ■ 5. False ■ 6. A. 25 ■ 7. B. 60 ■ 8. D. 19 ■ 9. B. 40 ■ 10. B. 40

Put a few drops of oregano oil in your moisturizer to kill surface bacteria and boost blood flow. Or, incorporate sage into your regimen. It regulates oil production, so it's the ultimate acne fighter, plus its calming effects work wonders for women going through menopause.

You may be thinking, "Sure, ancient civilizations used plants because that's all they had. Modern medicine is more targeted and sophisticated." However, plant-based compounds are used in many modern pharmaceuticals. Simply put, plants are natural healers. That fact hasn't changed since the beginning of time. It's only evolved across generations as it's merged with modern delivery systems and scientific tools.

Herbal Medicine Today

Today, more than three-quarters of the planet uses herbal medicine. Western researchers have proven in studies what generations have passed down for centuries: Plants grown and used at home are effective at treating *non-life-threatening* diseases and injuries or ailments such as bumps, bruises, headaches, fever, stress, depression, fatigue, and more.

It makes sense. Consider all the plants you eat on a regular basis (yep, the same ones you pull from your garden or the produce section of your favorite grocer): parsley, cilantro, sage, thyme, garlic, basil, ginger, mint. You might toss them in a garden salad because they add kicks of flavor, but those same herbs, spices, and, in some cases, vegetables, do double-duty once inside your body. They carry antioxidants and nutrients that bolster the immune system to fight disease before it starts. In modern doctors' circles, they call that "preventive" medicine. So why wouldn't those same herbs be used just as successfully for healing *after* you've gotten sick? St. John's Wort looks beautiful in a vase, but it's also fantastic for lowering stress. Chamomile makes a lovely after-dinner tea or you can use it to relieve indigestion, alleviate muscle spasms, reduce inflammation, or cure infections. Talk about getting two (or more) for one.

THE BENEFITS OF USING HERBAL MEDICINE

Nothing is more empowering than taking charge of your own health. Thanks to the power of herbal medicine, combined with your knowledge about the best ways to use it and the science of modern delivery systems, you're able to fully experience its benefits with safe, do-it-yourself methods in your own home. If you need more convincing, here are five compelling reasons to test-drive herbs yourself:

FOR HEAD, SHOULDERS, KNEES, AND TOES (AND NOSE)

The Skinny on Essential Oils & Aromatherapy

Aromatherapy products are incredibly popular now and getting ever more so. But wait a minute. Let's all take a deep breath, inhale the fragrances that surround us, and understand what the term means.

Aromatherapy involves the use of fragrant (aromatic) plant extracts, typically found in the essential oils of plants, with the intent to improve physical, mental, and emotional well-being. You can't enter a health food store, lifestyle store, clothes boutique, or home goods shop without finding an aisle of essential oil–based candles, incense, potpourri, soaps, lotions, or cleaners. And while you can light a scented candle to make your living room smell better, what makes an aromatherapy product truly, well, therapeutic, is when its use is not merely to please passively but to heal or help actively.

Aromatherapy practice is not limited to inhaling essential oils for their stimulating brain and mood effects, though that's a popular method. It also includes applying them topically so their healing molecules go to work in the bloodstream. What makes this practice so versatile (and cool) is that it's noninvasive so it can work solo or complementarily, alongside other alternative or mainstream remedies, or therapies, like a booster shot.

The Super Fuel Behind Aromatherapy

So what, exactly, are essential oils? Truly the super fuel behind aromatherapy, essential oils are highly concentrated, nutrient-dense compounds that are expelled, pressed, or extracted from plants. Think of them like the immune system of a plant, keeping it safe from pollutants, insects, and other toxins. Essential oils work the same way in your body. In the case of aromatherapy, they work via smell or absorption to heal the mind, body, and spirit. Unlike drugs that mask symptoms, essential oils work on the root causes of your issue so you deal with problems head-on and quickly rather than simply soothe their side effects.

In medical circles, these power-houses are called adaptogens, which are substances that work in a variety of ways to balance your body's systems, fight stress, and beat fatigue so you ward off disease and stay healthy. Studies show that adaptogens can do everything from speed healing to suppress infections without the side effects or downtime of some pharmaceuticals.

Some essential oils also do double duty as analgesics, which means they have the ability to reduce pain. Clove, birch, peppermint, and thyme are particularly effective analgesics. For instance, thyme essential oil has been shown in studies to alleviate menstrual pain better than ibuprofen, as well as inhibit COX-2, the enzyme that when overproduced in the body creates chronic inflammation and pain.

See chapters 8 (page 165) and 9 (page 191) for smelling salt recipes that rely on aromatherapy for mental and physical relief and well-being.

Knowing the Good From the Bad

Unfortunately, not all essential oils are created equal. And like most industries where business is booming, you'll find brands that don't live up to their hype.

Keep in mind that there's no authoritative body for essential oils that ensures quality, verifies ingredients, or regulates labeling terminology. On labels, you'll find all sorts of claims from "pure" and "therapeutic grade" to "all-natural" and "organic." While those sorts of marketing terms are essentially meaningless, there are ways to get the quality you need when prepping for DIY handcrafting. Look for labels that note "100 percent pure" oils, which are unadulterated and contain the optimal ratio of therapeutic compounds. Those that aren't labeled "100 percent pure" may be blends of other oils in order to market the product more expensively. It's like an "extra-virgin olive oil" that you discover is actually a blend of canola and olive oil when you read the ingredients. This distinction is important. These healing remedies are effective due to their complete botanical profile that works in unison both within the plant and later in your body to create healing results. When tampered or diluted, the benefits may be lessened or eliminated altogether.

Check out Resources (page 292) for a list of reliable brands. For more on shopping for the right essential oils, see chapter 2 (page 25).

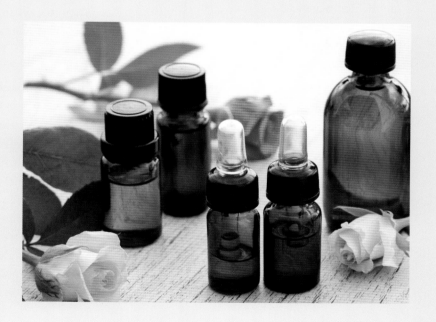

They're safe. For centuries, herbal medicine has used nontoxic herbs that are ingredients found in food, medicine, and beauty products. There's no guesswork about whether they're harmful. They're not. (Toxic herbs aren't for sale commercially.) If you experience any effects you didn't anticipate from using an herb, it's likely due to the amount taken—you've overindulged. Any discomfort is short term, the time it takes for the compounds to leave your system. One rule of thumb: If you're allergic to a plant, herb, or spice, you're allergic to its essential oils, too.

They're chemical-free. To be clear, not all herbal medicines are organic. However, most of the herbal remedies and essential oils in this book can be purchased organically, or if you're growing at home, you control the purity, quality, and care methods.

They're cheap. Hands down, homegrown herbs are more affordable than prescription meds, even with a copay! This benefit also applies to commercially sold herbal products, which can get pricey depending on the herb or where you shop (ahem, Whole Foods). Lavender essential oil, for instance, helps you fall asleep for pennies per snooze, which is far cheaper than comparable over-the-counter or prescription options.

They're readily available. The Internet and large grocery store and health food chains have made even the hardest-to-source herbs, essential oils, and seeds accessible for purchase. And, even if you don't have a garden or farm, your windowsill makes the perfect platform for growing potted herbs you can play with in the kitchen.

They're easy to work with. You don't need to be a botanist, herbalist, scientist, or any other "ist" for successful DIY herbal medicine. You don't even need to have a green thumb. Most plants that fall into the category of "medicinal" are also considered "weedy." Weeds by nature are almost impossible to get rid of. They're sturdy, hardy survivalists. That's why they're easy to grow, they thrive in harsh conditions, and their "never say die" constitution works just as hard in your body.

You'll see from reading this book that there aren't many treatments or remedies more versatile than herbal medicine. While you might pop a prescription Ambien when you need to sleep, you won't rub it on a wound to make it

TREAT YOURSELF

HIGH-QUALITY LABELS AND A SHARPIE

No matter how photographic your memory, the bigger your herbal medicine cabinet becomes, the harder it is to track its contents, especially when it all starts looking the same. Each label should include the name, ingredients, dosage, and date prepared.

heal faster. Or, you might suck on a lozenge to ease throat pain but it won't do much for a back spasm. The opposite's true of plant-based compounds. They're extremely versatile and thanks to a variety of delivery systems—tinctures, teas, lotions, shampoos, massage oils, candles, and more—they're used to prevent or treat more than one issue, especially when used in combination with other herbs. For instance, your everyday garlic bulb can be pickled and eaten to fight colds and flu, combined with olive oil to heal ear infections, or mixed with an herb blend and oil to ease digestion. Aloe vera is another great example. It can be added to lotion for its anti-aging properties, combined with herbs and oils to heal burns, or rubbed over arthritic areas to ease inflammation and pain.

Throughout this book, we'll cover the top herbs and their multitude of uses in a variety of areas: body (for cosmetic, wellness, and healing purposes); mental health (for stress, anxiety, depression, and more); nontoxic home care products (everything from candles to cleaners); and "morning afters."

HERBAL MEDICINE GOES MAINSTREAM

Herbal medicine still thrives throughout the world as researchers prove it's both effective and safe as alternative and complementary solutions to costly prescriptions and expensive treatments. Forecasters expect the global market for supplements and herbs to top $107 billion by 2017.

Herbalists are no longer only gardeners, farmers, or botanists. You'll find herb experts around the world working in a variety of practices. They're Traditional Chinese Medicine doctors, medical doctors, naturopaths, osteopaths, acupuncturists, chiropractors, pharmacists, compounding pharmacists, registered dieticians, estheticians, and more. And, thanks to modern transportation and packaging systems, you're no longer reliant on what's seasonal or local in your at-home healing practice. Herbs grown natively in Thailand, Peru, India, or New Zealand are readily available online, in your local health food store, or, yes, even grown on your own windowsill.

YOU DON'T NEED TO BE A BOTANIST, HERBALIST, SCIENTIST, OR ANY OTHER "IST" TO MAKE DIY HERBAL MEDICINE

JUST LIKE US

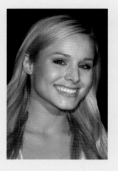

THE CELEB: Kristen Bell

THE HERBS: coconut oil and essential oils of black pepper, clary sage, bergamot, tea tree, and grapefruit

THE USES: Body scrub and deodorant

WHETHER YOU LOVED HER as Veronica Mars, or your daughter idolizes her as the spirited Princess Anna from the movie *Frozen*, Kristen has been capturing our attention for years with her beauty, wit, humor, and singing chops. When it comes to her skin, you'd imagine that Kristen could purchase any product she desires. Instead, she makes her own simple body scrub from brown sugar, honey, and coconut oil. And to help stay fresh through long days on set, her go-to deodorant is an aluminum-free cream ($12) from the herbal body care company Fat and the Moon. Essential oils make up five of the cream's nine ingredients, ensuring a potent, fragrant, and health-conscious alternative for women everywhere.

Naturopathy Meets Western Medicine

Naturopaths—those who make use of natural herbs and remedies in their medicinal approaches—have been practicing herbal medicine formally for a range of conditions since the turn of the twentieth century. While this might seem "alternative" in the United States, other parts of the world have a more integrated philosophy of medicine. An article published by the University of Maryland Medical Center estimates that, in Germany, 70 percent of physicians prescribe nearly 700 plant-based medicines in their practices.

But the United States is catching up. Greater numbers of medical doctors than ever before are working in conjunction with naturopathic doctors and herbalists to put together treatment plans that incorporate herbs into medical protocols. According to Gabrielle Francis, a naturopathic physician, chiropractor, and licensed acupuncturist based in New York City, the best example of the complementary use of herbs and Western medicine is currently happening at the Cancer Treatment Centers of America. Many herbal remedies are administered during chemotherapy and radiation treatments to reduce side effects such as nausea, ulcers, and wasting syndrome. In the weeks after chemotherapy and radiation ends, herbal remedies help to detox the medications out of the body. As reported in the *Wall Street Journal*, a study partially funded by the National Cancer Institute confirms that *huang qin tang*—an herb that practitioners of traditional Chinese medicine have used for centuries—does reduce the side effects of chemotherapy, as well as enhances colon cancer treatment. Researchers have isolated sixty-two individual active ingredients in the single herb that work together to treat the disease.

At the Yale University School of Medicine, Dr. Yung Chi Cheng has carved out a name for himself by publishing and speaking on the significant contributions of herbal medicine to pharmacological research. His studies of Chinese herbs in combination with Western medicine have led to innovative therapies for hard-to-treat diseases such as HIV/AIDS and hepatitis B.

Yale isn't the only hotbed of integrative medical research. Kathi Kemper, MD, is director for the Center for Integrative Health and Wellness at Ohio State University, and has been integrating mind-body therapies with Western medicine since 1981. She offers a formal curriculum to teach doctors-in-training alternative practices such as hypnosis, guided imagery, and meditation to enhance their personal lives, their practice, and their patients' outcomes. In addition, she's conducted numerous studies and interviews supporting the use of herbal medicine in treating ailments like ADD (attention deficit disorder)/ADHD (attention deficit hyperactivity disorder), allergies, colds, depression, and headaches.

In her naturopathic practice, Dr. Francis reports that she has seen great results in treating the following conditions with their corresponding herbal preparations:

- **Leaky gut syndrome:** aloe vera, licorice, marshmallow, and slippery elm
- **Parasites and candida:** peppermint, oregano, thyme, goldenseal, wormwood, black walnut, and berberine
- **Adrenal fatigue:** licorice, Siberian ginseng, and rhodiola
- **Fertility:** vitex

Dr. Francis notes that, while certain preparations are best for specific conditions, it's important to remember that at the very least, herbs can be used as nutritional support in the same way that food is medicine. "Herbs provide vitamins, minerals, electrolytes, and other food-like compounds that have a building effect in the body," she says. On days when you feel more like cooking than making a salve, herbs can still work their magic through teas, stews, salads, and other everyday kitchen creations.

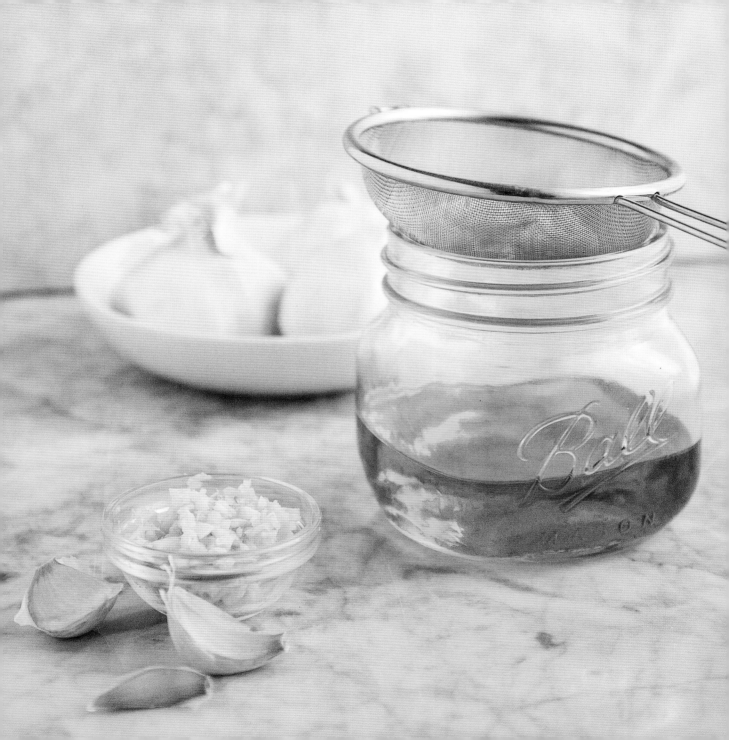

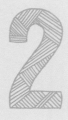

THE HERBAL WORKSHOP

Techniques and Tools

Now that you've got the lowdown on the benefits and ease of at-home herbal medicine, it's time to get your space stocked and set up for some simple preparations. While it's tempting to go full-on DIY, that's not practical—or necessary. You can get a lot of bang for little buck by starting simple, investing in the right equipment, and using minimal ingredients that are as versatile as they are healthy.

STARTING AN INDOOR MEDICINAL HERB GARDEN

No need to go crazy with high-tech greenhouse lighting, innovative irrigation systems, or expensive seeds, soil, or containers. Remember, this is low-maintenance gardening for the easy-going DIYer who doesn't want to break the bank. Planting can be done in three super-simple steps . . . ready, set, grow!

1. **Choose your container.** Unless you're a seasoned crafter and want to build your own, stop by a gardening store and buy something that fits into your style and décor. Must haves? The pot should stand at least 6 to 8 inches tall, have drainage at the bottom, and come with a tray to prevent water leakage from damaging your sill or furniture.

2. **Pick your soil.** The better the dirt, the better your garden will grow. Look for fast-draining varieties that you can mix with your favorite secret fertilizing weapon: sand, coffee grounds, lime peels—whatever you use to nourish your house plants will work here, too (except chemical sprays, of course).

3. **Plant your herbs.** Start with just three to four herbs (remember, you're not farming, you're prepping a simple indoor garden) and shoot for the most versatile types, like basil, mint, ginger, thyme, sage, garlic, or echinacea. While you may be tempted to use seeds, which are inexpensive, they can take two to three weeks to grow, whereas seedlings or full-on plants will be ready much sooner.

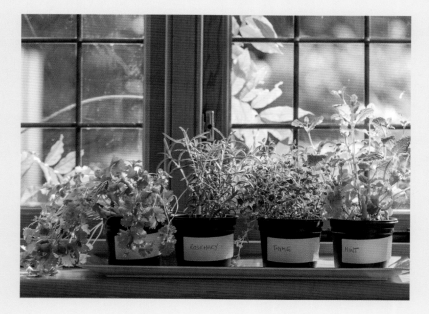

The fastest, easiest way to begin is with a small garden, whether it's in your yard or on a countertop. Doing so connects you to the source of your healing and empowers you to take as much care of your herbs as you do your mind, body, and spirit. If you've already got a garden, life just got even easier. Medicinal herbs are a cinch to incorporate into plots or planters you've already got growing.

Next you'll need to identify the types of herbal preparations that appeal to you, anything from tinctures to teas and everything in between. This book will help you choose the right herbs for yourself and the best ways to prepare them for your needs and lifestyle.

No worries if you're not a master chef or have a love-hate relationship with your kitchen. Making herbal remedies doesn't require any specific skills or talents, rather a genuine interest in your health and a little time. The good news is that you really can't mess it up as long as you follow the simple instructions.

This chapter is your step-by-step guide to understanding the tools and techniques you need to create a one-of-a-kind "pharmacy." By the end, you'll be ready to make lotions, shampoos, teas, salves, tinctures, baths, syrups, home-cleaning products, and more (see The Remedies, page 95). Beginners, fear not. This is as much fun as it is easy!

HERBAL PREPARATIONS

After growing or purchasing the herbs that appeal to you, you'll be ready to begin making preparations. Each preparation has its own function and targets specific issues and concerns, but is not plant-specific, meaning you can mix and match your concoctions with different methods.

On the following pages, you'll find preparations divided into two sections: **Preparations for Health and Wellness** and **Preparations for Cosmetic Care**. Each section aims to educate you about the herbal approach, and includes application methods, the kitchen equipment you'll need to create them, and the storage containers you'll want to have on hand. Preceding the section on cosmetic care preparations is a **Know Your Skin** guide to help you determine which treatments will work best with your skin type.

HERBAL TEAS

Herbal tea is a bit of a misnomer because it's not technically a tea. A *tea* by definition is a drink made by steeping the cured leaves of the specific tea plant (*Camellia sinensis*) in hot water and includes varieties such as oolong, black, white, yellow, and green. *Herbal tea* on the other hand is a blend of herbs, spices, and just about anything else you'd get from a plant steeped in hot or boiling water. You can use roots, bark, flowers, peels, fruit, chunks of lemon or ginger—add to your own list. Red tea, a.k.a. rooibos, also falls into the herbal category despite its name. One way to think about it is that herbal teas are made from most anything you'd find in the garden, like chamomile, mint, and echinacea.

While most of the world is fairly particular about drinking only the "true" teas, the United States is obsessed with herbal teas (thanks to their antioxidant levels, medicinal uses, and lack of caffeine) and doesn't seem to mind the misnomer. Keeping this in mind, this book uses the term *tea* generically.

Once you understand the difference between herbal and non-herbal teas, the next thing to know is that there are two types of herbal teas: infusions and decoctions.

Infusion

An *infusion* is a tea made by pouring boiling water over delicate parts of the plant—like fruits, leaves, dried flowers, berries, or buds—and then steeping the liquid so the nutrients are imparted into the drink. This practice is different from cooking the tea in a pot over heat, which destroys nutrients and enzymes. Instead, you'll gently let the steeping tea "free float" in a jar to maximize extraction. This method allows you to get both the flavors and the nutrients from the herbs. You can use dried herbs as well as fresh ones. Just be sure that the dried herbs haven't passed their shelf life, which diminishes their healing power and potency. Once the herbs are strained off, your infusion is ready to drink. A French press is a handy way to create infusions.

Tea infusions are used for their flavor or medicinal purposes or both. They're a great way to incorporate herbs on an everyday basis.

Application method: Aromatic, internal, topical (poultice or compress)

Kitchen equipment: Pan, lidded jars, French press (optional)

Storage equipment: Lidded jars or tins (for extra herb blend); lidded jars or pitchers to store extra infusions

Decoction

While infusions are made from the most delicate parts of plants, *decoctions* are high-powered herbal teas made from the hardiest parts of plants, such as fibrous stems, thick bark, seeds, nuts, or roots. Because these components tend to be on the rougher, denser side, it takes a slow heat to extract all their minerals and healing elements. In other words, simply steeping them in boiling water isn't enough to release the potent nutrients and the richer flavors inside these hardier, tougher mixtures.

Decoctions require that you combine all of your herbs into a non-aluminum pot with cold water and slowly bring the mixture to a boil. (Avoid aluminum because it might cause a chemical reaction with some herbs.) There's no set time limit on how long to simmer or boil. Instead, wait until the water reduces by two-thirds of its original amount, leaving an extraordinarily concentrated medicinal drink. Strain off the herb mixture before you drink the remaining decoction.

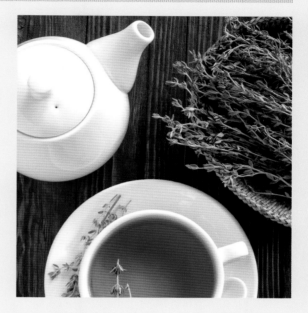

Application method: Aromatic, internal, topical (poultice or compress)

Kitchen equipment: Pan, strainer

Storage equipment: Lidded jars or tins (for extra herb blend); lidded jars or pitchers to store extra decoction

OILS

If you've made salad dressing or chili oil for bread dipping, then you've basically made an herbal oil. The only difference with the method described here is you'll heat the oil and use herbs designed to target specific health issues. While there's a recent explosion of herbal oils in the marketplace—such as rosemary for hair and scalp, and calendula for skin ailments—they're not a new thing. In fact, they've been used for centuries to impart the healing nutrients of plants into the skin. The types you'll use in this book aren't any different than the ones you'll find in a high-end spa treatment room or on department store shelves, except the price tag is much lower.

Olive oil is the go-to oil for herbal medicine because it's chock full of healthy fatty acids. Its viscosity makes it perfect for massaging into skin and prepping salves, too. Because it has a faint olive smell, you may not love it for bath oils, but it does the trick in terms of nourishing and moisturizing your skin.

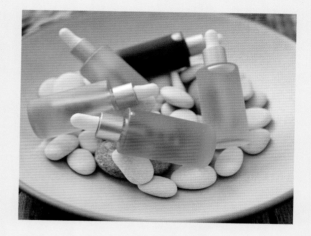

Regardless of which herbal remedies you prepare, start with a carrier oil. Carrier oils are used to dilute highly concentrated essential oils before they're applied to your body.

Application method: Aromatic, internal, topical

Kitchen equipment: Double boiler or a saucepan with a stainless steel bowl atop, stainless steel strainer, cheesecloth

Storage equipment: Glass jars, labels

SALVES AND BALMS

Salves and *balms* are ointments designed to heal, protect, or soothe the skin. The basic ingredient is generally a carrier oil, an essential oil or infused oil (carrier oil spiked with healing herbs), beeswax, or some combo of oils and waxes as their foundation. From here, choose your ingredients based on the issues you're trying to treat, such as rashes, acne, dry skin, chapped lips, bug bites, allergies, sunburn, and more. Most of the herbs you'll need are easily found in your backyard or on your windowsill and are teeming with skin-fixing nutrients and essential oils. Or, skip a step and start with infused oils so you have less doctoring up to do.

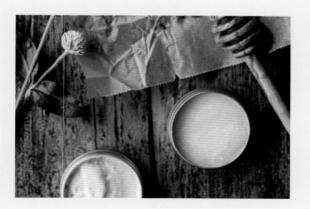

Most herbalists, naturopaths, aromatherapists, and alternative medicine experts use the terms "salve" and "balm" interchangeably. Both preparations can vary in thickness and ratio of oils to wax based on your personal preference and application needs. However, they should contain zero waters or fats, both of which are reserved for preparing lotions and creams. Salves and balms are designed to be placed topically on the skin as a vehicle for imparting healing components into your body.

Application method: Aromatic, topical

Kitchen equipment: Double boiler or a saucepan with a stainless steel bowl atop, stainless steel strainer, cheesecloth

Storage equipment: Glass jars or tins, labels

TINCTURES AND LINIMENTS

A *tincture* is the concentrated liquid form of an herb that is taken orally or used as an external remedy. Tinctures are made by soaking herbs in a solvent—basically, a substance that dissolves other substances to form a solution. Alcohols such as vodka and gin are the most common solvents used in tinctures, though apple cider vinegar is another option that is growing in popularity. The solvent works by extracting the essential compounds from the herb. The mixture is then strained and transferred to a dark bottle.

Alcohols used in tinctures should be in the 80- to 100-proof range for maximum extraction of herbal nutrients, essential oils, and other healing plant juices. Eighty to 90-proof alcohols also work if you're using non-juicy or dried herbs in your tincture. Many herbalists believe that if the concentration is made with anything other than alcohol, it's not a tincture, rather an *extract*.

A *liniment* is a type of tincture that is applied topically, not internally. This book does not include any remedies, other than teas, for oral ingestion.

Application method: Internal, topical

Kitchen equipment: Knife, cutting board, alcohol, glass jar with lid

Storage equipment: Dark glass bottle with a dropper

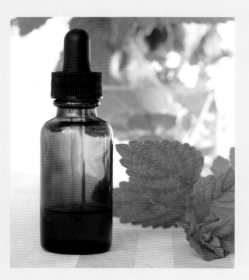

BATHS

Baths are like herbal teas for your body. Depending on the types of herbs you use and the temperature of your water, your preparation can stimulate your senses or relax them. For example, herbs like chamomile or rosemary are perfect for nighttime relaxation, while peppermint and green tea make for amazing morning pick-me-ups. Herbal baths can produce great healing results. They increase circulation, soothe aching muscles, lower stress, stave off colds and flu, relieve inflammation, boost the mood, tone the skin, and promote cell repair. Basically, herbal baths are limited only by their specific therapeutic healing powers. You may be surprised to know how beneficial bathing can be with simply the herbs you've got stashed in your refrigerator's crisper.

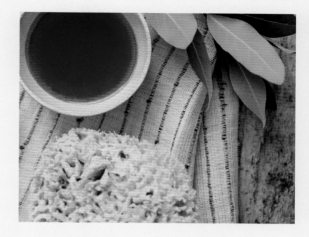

How do these herbs work in the bath? Like steam in a facial, bath water opens pores in your skin, which allows the healing compounds you're soaking in to seep into your body. Your herbal body tea is more than enough to provide ample healing. However, you can take the experience up a notch by dimming the lights and adding candles.

Application method: Aromatic, topical

Kitchen equipment: Cheesecloth, or strainer (a handkerchief or nylon stocking will also work)

Storage equipment: Jar with lid

POULTICES AND COMPRESSES

A *poultice* is fresh or dried plant parts, usually warmed, and placed in a piece of cloth to be used like a bandage. Poultices are applied to wounds and inflammation to stop pain, swelling, and soreness.

A *compress* is a piece of cloth that is soaked in herbs and then applied damp to the affected part of the body. It can be any temperature depending on how it's used.

Compresses and poultices have been used in various forms as antiseptics and anti-inflammatories. At their heart, both techniques involve placing wet or moist herbs over a physical problem area so the skin tissue absorbs the herbal therapies. They've been in play since the early days of China, Egypt, and Greece.

Poultices

Poultices are simply a combination of moist herbs, clay, or other absorbent substances applied directly to the skin or affected areas. You choose the herb or herbal blend based on your particular ailment, while the herbs or clay act as an absorbent, rather than a nutrient, so use whatever you have available. This warm paste-like remedy is then placed over your wound and kept warm with a heating pad or towel to reduce inflammation and draw out infection if there is any. Generally, poultices are left on until the clay dries out, or until the poultice is cooled and the ailment reevaluated.

If you've got burns, bites, rashes, achy muscles, pimples or blemishes, tumors, cysts, swollen glands, sprains, or similar conditions in which you need to draw out impurities, boost circulation to an area, or soothe irritation, this is your go-to treatment.

Application method: Aromatic, topical

Kitchen equipment: Cotton fabrics (optional)

Storage equipment: n/a

Compresses

A compress is similar to a poultice in that you're drawing out impurities and increasing circulation to a problem area. However, unlike a poultice, this remedy is simply about applying a hot or cold liquid onto your skin via a towel (rather than a paste made entirely of herbs).

Where do the herbs come into play? Instead of a traditional compress of water, you'll use an herbal tea or essential oil in water as your liquid.

Compresses are typically easier to make and prepare compared to poultices. This is particularly the case if you're already brewing a pot of herbal tea. The only real downside to both these preparations is that they can be messy to create and use, which limits their portability and functionality.

To reduce swelling and inflammation, use cold compresses for 45 to 60 minutes at a time throughout the day. Cold compresses are good for treating bruises, swollen glands, sunburns, sprains, aches and pains, digestive issues, skin issues, respiratory problems, constipation, and even irritable bowel syndrome.

Hot compresses move blood to your skin's surface, which helps get impurities out of your system. For example, they can help alleviate the discomfort of congestion. Simply place the treated towel on your face to receive some relief.

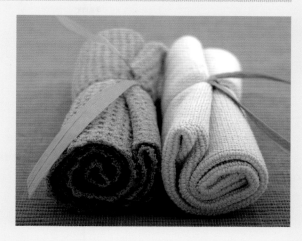

Application method: Aromatic, topical

Kitchen equipment: Soft cotton fabric towels

Storage equipment: n/a

KNOW YOUR SKIN

Connect your skin type to the appropriate care to kick start home-based treatments that'll have your skin glowing.

You wouldn't buy facial moisturizers or cleansers without knowing your skin type. Same thing goes for herbal medicine. Before you can effectively treat your body with plant-based creams and soaps, it's important to know which of these five characteristics best describes your skin:

Normal or Balanced ▪ Oily ▪ Dry ▪ Combination ▪ Sensitive

This knowledge allows you to manage the ingredients that go into your preparations, and their ratios, for optimal efficacy. Plus, it's the key to flawless-looking skin. Check out this breakdown and be sure to reassess your skin's condition every few months as it changes with seasons, hormones, weather, and stress levels:

Normal or Balanced

Normal or *balanced* skin is exactly like the name implies: neither too oily nor too dry. It's got few to zero imperfections or blemishes, barely visible pores, little to no sensitivity, and a beautifully glowing radiance. Yep, you guessed it...this is the skin people strive for. The only issues you may experience are the occasional blackheads in the T zone (chin, nose, forehead) or upper back, along with head-to-toe dehydration in the winter—nothing that drinking water and applying lotion can't fix.

CARE: Opt for gentle, water-based soaps, lotion-like cleansers, cleansing oils or oat-, nut-, or seed-based milk or clay blends for both face and body. For post-cleansing, mist tea- or herbal vinegar–based toner over skin—for example, rose, calendula, chamomile, rosemary, or lavender—followed by a lightweight moisturizer to lock-in hydration.

Oily

If you've got medium to large pores in your T zone, back, chest, neck, or shoulders, you're likely *oily*. This type of skin is often shiny again just an hour post-cleansing, and makeup tends to vanish quickly after application. While you might be acne-prone, the upside is that well-hydrated skin tends to have zero fine lines and very few wrinkles.

CARE: Twice daily, use a gentle, moisturizing soap, gel, or cleanser. It should be water-, milk-, or clay-based and can include finely ground nuts, seeds, and oats to aid in hydration. It sounds counterintuitive but dehydrated skin makes oil worse, because lack of moisture triggers the skin glands to produce a fatty secretion (called sebum) to compensate, which results in oilier skin. Follow your soap or cleanser with hydrating mist, lightweight herbal moisturizers, and twice-weekly scrubs or masks to keep oil at bay.

Dry

While *dry* skin has small pores, it lacks the moisture necessary to create a flawless, radiant glow. Signs you've got dryness? Flakiness, red irritated patches, fine lines, wrinkles, and a tight feeling, especially after cleansing.

CARE: Avoid dehydrating skin further by swapping out soap for creamy, moisturizing cleansing lotions or oil-based cleansers as your face wash. Soothe irritation and dial-up moisture with a toner or splash made with herbal teas. Lemon balm, fennel, neroli, lavender, marshmallow root, or calendula are some good candidates. Hydrate head to toe with an ultra-lush moisturizer designed to heal, repair, and nourish skin.

Combination

Combination skin gets its name for a reason: You've got a combination of multiple skin types, say oily in the T zone with dryness in the cheeks. This means you're likely prone to flakiness in certain areas and breakouts in others, and as a general rule, skin is sensitive.

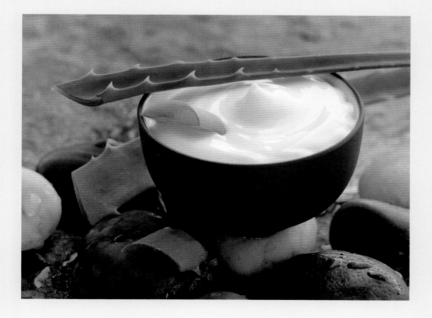

CARE: This type needs extra love! Cleanse head to toe with products designed to treat oily skin (gentle, moisturizing cleansing lotions, oils, or lathers). Tone face with a mild herb-infused apple cider vinegar (try rose, comfrey, lavender, or chamomile). The same herb blend can be used to create a tea-based body wash for post-shower. Hydrate with a light- or medium-weight moisturizer or add a few drops of herbal tincture to your favorite lotions.

Sensitive

Sensitive skin reacts strongly to external conditions, such as weather, temperature, skin care products or ingredients, foods, and more. If you're the type that burns easily in the sun, gets rashes or irritation when exposed to particular elements, or experiences redness when air is too hot, cold, dry, or humid, this skin type might be yours.

CARE: Treat delicate skin like you would oily skin with the exception of cleansing tools. Never use harsh brushes, thick or knobby towels, loofahs, sponges, or exfoliating tools on a sensitive face.

FACIAL CLEANSERS

Facial cleansers are made by melting solids, such as shea butter, cocoa butter, or beeswax, so they're better able to mix with essential or infused oils. The type of butter or wax you use depends on whether you want a creamier, thicker, or firmer consistency. There's no magic thickness or right texture—it's simply a matter of your personal preference. You can store your end products in the bathroom with your other skincare supplies and they'll last 30 days or so. Remember, they've got no preservatives! To stretch the shelf life, keep your cleanser unopened in the refrigerator and it will stay fresh for up to six months.

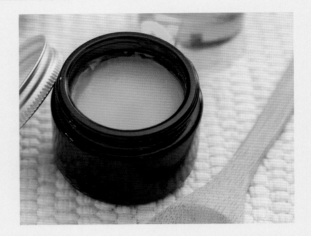

Skin type: All

Kitchen equipment: Double boiler or a saucepan with a stainless steel bowl atop

Storage equipment: Plastic or glass jars or bottles

TONERS AND ASTRINGENTS

A *toner* is a lotion or wash designed to brighten and refresh sensitive, dry, or normal skin types. They can be used to cleanse the skin and shrink the appearance of pores, and are usually used on the face.

Astringents are more powerful forms of toners, particularly commercial varieties, which are often made with isopropyl alcohol or acetone (yeah, that same stuff that's in your nail polish), so you can imagine how drying and harsh it is to skin. The bonus of herbal astringents is that they're soothing and gentle, but still effective.

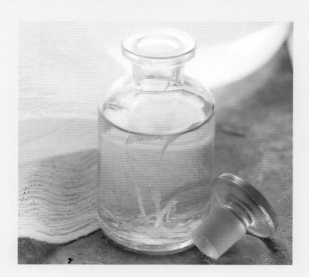

The main purpose of astringents and toners is to wipe skin of residual cleansers, dirt, or oil. They also prep skin for moisturizer and balance *pH levels* while also tightening tissue, reducing swelling, and easing inflammation. Most astringents and toners in the recipes in Part 3 (page 95) contain alcohol-free witch hazel extract, a powerful but simple ingredient for pulling impurities from the skin.

While astringents and toners do not have to be refrigerated, applying them cold shrinks tissues more effectively than at room temperature, plus it feels great on a hot day. Guarantee freshness by storing them in tightly lidded glass bottles, spritzers, or jars. Make sure you've got cotton squares on hand to apply the solution on the face and neck in upward, outward strokes.

Skin type: Astringents: Combination, Normal, Oily; Toners: Dry, Normal, Sensitive

Kitchen equipment: n/a

Storage equipment: Storage containers, bottles or jars with lids, or spray bottles

MASKS

A *mask* is simply a skin treatment used for detoxing, deep cleaning, and purifying skin, head to toe. Masks are one of the oldest beauty secrets (you can thank the ancient Egyptians for this one). While masks used to be primarily made of clay, modern DIYers are also using grains, fruit or vegetable mashes, aloe vera, and more to get flawless, radiant, deep-clean skin.

The beauty behind this treatment is that you can customize your mask to your particular skin needs to do far more than sweep pores of dirt and grime. Depending on the herbs you blend, today's "high-tech" all-natural preparation can soothe irritation, rid your system of toxins, amp up circulation, calm inflammation, tighten pores, replenish moisture, and brighten your look. Not bad for something that takes minutes to prep with stuff you find in your garden or crisper.

See individual recipes for specific application and preparation guidelines. For the most part, you can make masks easily and quickly. Simply whisk ingredients into a paste in a bowl before applying to your face or other part of the body. Then relax while the mask does

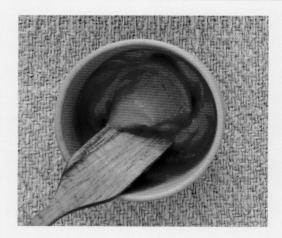

its thing. Remove with your fingertips. Recipes tend to be gentle enough for weekly or semiweekly use, but you know your skin, so you be the judge.

Skin type: All

Kitchen equipment: Bowls, whisk, spoon

Storage equipment: Most masks are intended for a single treatment but dry ingredients can be stored in a plastic or glass jar, zip-seal plastic bag, or a tin.

MOISTURIZERS

A *moisturizer* is a preparation that hydrates your cells. It acts like a protective shield that separates your skin from the harsh elements including weather, seasonal changes, pollutants, dirt, and more. These formulas can be made in different weights (light to thick), using oil or water bases, so you can customize them according to whether you need more or less hydration. Generally speaking, you'll apply ½ to 1 teaspoon over your entire face after cleansing, toning, or applying a scrub or mask.

You'll see that some of the recipes in this book require cooking the ingredients in a double boiler over low heat, to melt solids like beeswax or cocoa butter, and others require no more than whisking ingredients in a bowl. The common thread in all of the recipes? You'll see amazing results in a very short time with minimal effort—certainly no more than making a quick stovetop meal.

These beauties have a shelf life of about one month. Moisturizers need no refrigeration, making them perfect to store along with your other skincare products. If you refrigerate in a tightly sealed container in the fridge, the formulas can last up to six months.

Skin type: All

Kitchen equipment: Double boiler or a saucepan with a stainless steel bowl atop, small bowl, whisk

Storage equipment: Glass jar

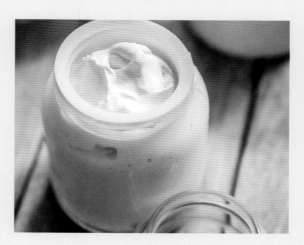

SCRUBS

Scrubs are designed to slough off dead, dry cells from your skin's surface, leaving it softer, smoother, and more radiant. Use daily or weekly, and over time you'll speed cell turnover, smooth complexion, even skin tone, and brighten your glow—all the same promises you get from a $200 jar of luxury skincare but without the chemicals and high price tag.

If you're a connoisseur of commercial brands, you're likely familiar with their rough granular texture and harsh ingredients. The recipes in this book are softer and gentler so you're guaranteed smoother, more nourishing results. In fact, unlike chemical- and preservative-laden store brands, these blends don't strip skin of its natural oils, so you can safely use them as your daily face wash, especially if you wear little to no makeup.

The key with scrubs is that you're letting the product do the "scrubbing," not your hands. The skin on your face and neck is far too gentle for you to rub in the product or exfoliate it the way you would elbows, knees, and feet. Instead, slather on gently—avoiding the ultrasensitive eye area—and let it go to work. Leave on 15 to 20 minutes before rinsing.

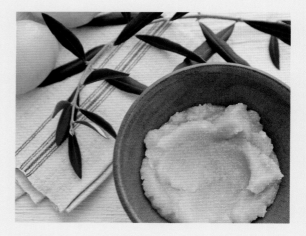

Skin type: All skin types except ones currently experiencing acne, broken veins, sensitivity, inflammation, irritation, sunburn, windburn, or rosacea

Kitchen equipment: Double boiler or a saucepan with a stainless steel bowl atop, bowl, whisk

Storage equipment: Plastic or glass jars, zip-seal plastic bags. Dry ingredients can be stored in those same containers as well as tins.

SHOPPING FOR INGREDIENTS

You're now in the know about what you need to prepare, so it's time to shop! Most of the items you'll need can be found at your neighborhood home goods, hardware, or general merchandise stores. Alternatively, they're readily available online with the click of a few buttons. Nothing on these pages is extravagant, gourmet, or impossible to source.

Basic Kitchen Tools

Find these basics and you're on track for creating a DIY herbal medicine workshop in a snap:

- double-meshed stainless steel strainer
- double boiler, or a medium saucepan and a slightly larger stainless steel bowl to perch on top
- glass jars with tight-fitting lids (such as Mason jars) and with spray tops, 4-ounce and 8-ounce
- dark glass bottle with a dropper for serum, 2-ounce, for toner (optional)
- tin containers with lids for salves and balms, 4-ounce and 8-ounce
- glass bowls in small, medium, and large

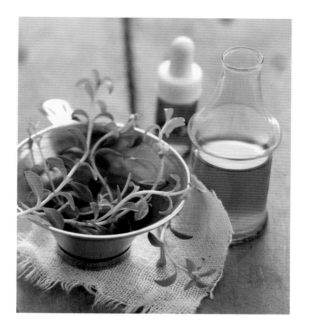

- measuring cups and spoons
- funnels
- grater (for beeswax and spices)
- cheesecloth
- labels to note a remedy and date
- a coffee grinder (or mini food processor) that has been thoroughly cleaned, or is purchased expressly for your herbal preparations

JUST LIKE US

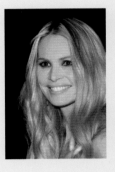

THE CELEB: Elle Macpherson

THE HERBS: Greens, Chinese herbs, medicinal mushrooms

THE USES: Migraines, exhaustion, and seasonal affective disorder

AS A SUPERMODEL and actress, Elle Macpherson is in a world of her own, in many regards. But Elle's choices for staying healthy and balanced are ones we can make for ourselves too: exercising regularly, observing a meat-free diet, and (here's the toughie) swearing off alcohol and aspirin. Elle has commented that, as an Australian, she's long been open to alternative medicines and homeopathic treatments for health and beauty. Her herbal regimen involves drinking blends of super greens, digestive enzymes, immune-boosting mushrooms, and Chinese herbs. With the goal of balancing stress, boosting skin radiance, and building immunity, Elle's herbal approach seems equally suited for supermodels, supermoms, and superwomen of any age.

Key Ingredients

No matter how you slice it, you'll be using some combination of the following ingredients: carrier oils, essential oils, and dried herbs. Read on to find out what you need to know about shopping for each.

Carrier Oils

Also known as "fixed" or "natural base" oils, the sole purpose of carrier oils in your herbal medicine lab is to dilute or stretch essential oils. They're made from seeds, nuts, and vegetables, and if you've ever gotten a professional massage, you've probably come into contact with one (or more). Or, if you've ever made a salad or pasta at home, you've got one or two in your pantry. The most common carrier oils for herbal preparations include the following:

- aloe vera oil
- olive oil
- jojoba oil
- grape seed oil
- walnut oil
- avocado oil
- sesame oil
- walnut oil
- almond oil

Carrier oils also make fantastic vehicles for aromatherapy blends and hydrating beauty treatments, as well as treating particular skin conditions, such as callouses, fungal infections, and even diaper rash. Because they're also rich in their own nutrients, vitamins, fatty acids, and minerals, each nourishes the skin in its own very specific way while imparting the healing compounds of the essential oils you blend with it.

All oils should be stored in cool, dark spaces like pantries and cupboards, and will last anywhere from six months to years. Check the individual label on each of the products you buy to make sure your particular carrier oil is fresh when you use it. In summer months, move carrier oils to the refrigerator if temperatures get too high to ensure safety and freshness. Many of them thicken or become solid like soft butter when chilled. So, remove them 12 hours before using so they thin back out and settle to room temperature.

Note: If you have nut allergies, steer clear of nut-based oils.

Essential Oils

Similar to food, skincare, medicine, and other products, ingredient lists are key to knowing if an essential oil lives up to its label's marketing claims in terms of purity and quality. Check out Resources (page 292) for the most reputable essential oil retailers. Before you buy, keep this checklist on hand:

Be a price tag detective. If you're eyeing a certain brand, look at the cost of the different oils the vendor offers in their product line. Variances reflect the fact that certain extracts will dictate different production costs. If the prices don't vary, that's a red flag that the manufacturer may be using inferior product or misrepresenting what's inside the bottle.

Choose dark bottles. High-quality essential oils are packed in green, amber, blue, or violet bottles, rather than clear, and typically with orifice reducers, not droppers which are often made with a rubber rim that can corrode oil. The dark colors help protect ingredients that are sensitive to light.

Pay attention to marketing lingo. You will see terms like "therapeutic" or "aromatherapy-grade" on essential oil bottles. Essential oil is not regulated by the FDA or any other authoritative

---

TREAT YOURSELF
TO A STYLISH AROMATHERAPY DIFFUSER

The ultimate desk (and health) accessory, purchasing a dispenser in a style you love ensures you set it out and reminds you to use it. Fill it with essential oils that increase productivity, ease stress, and energize you day in and day out.

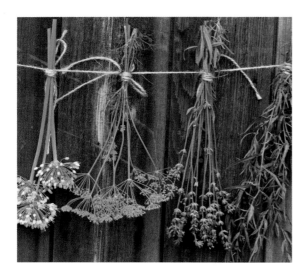

body. The important factors for you to take into consideration are:

- Has the product undergone gas chromatography–mass spectrometry (GC-MS) testing? It should have.
- Is the herb's Latin name on the bottle? It should be.
- Is the price lower than what other brands charge for the same oil? That's a red flag.
- What do real users have to say about the product or brand? Online reviews are excellent sources of information, particularly those posted on blogs. If you live near an independent store that sells essential oils, talk to sales staff. They tend to be extremely knowledgeable about their inventory.

Buy what's right for you. You know your body and what issues you're trying to treat. That's your focus when buying essential oils. Also, steer clear of your personal allergens. (Allergic to ginger? You're probably allergic to its essential oil.) Lastly, shopping by recipe is a fab way to start and branch out from the ingredient list as you build your medicine cabinet.

Fresh and Dried Herbs

The trick with both fresh and dried herbs is knowing what to buy before you shop. You want herbs that have a wide range of medicinal, fragrant, cleansing, nutritional, and flavoring uses. (In the same way you don't want to buy a spice cabinet full of expensive hard-to-source brands to make one exotic dish, you want your herbs to serve multiple purposes, too.) Also be sure to understand each herb's unique storage needs and shelf life so you use it at its peak freshness. Finally, buy organic to ensure the chemicals used in growing the herbs don't end up in or on your body.

Drying Fresh Herbs. If you've got access to a farm, backyard, or windowsill fresh herbs, it's super simple to dry them on your own before using them.

Pick or purchase herbs as they're becoming "ripe" (i.e., buds should be newly opened or just formed). If you're selecting herbs from outside make sure they are dirt-, chemical-, and moisture-free, and patted dry with a paper towel.

Set out a single layer of herbs in a well-ventilated, dimly lit area between 65 and 85 degrees Fahrenheit. You can place them on a countertop or on metal or mesh screen or netting, or hang them in 10-stem bundles from the stems. Drying takes three days to three weeks. Note: If you're drying a bunch of herbs at the same time, separate and label the paper towels because once dried, it will be tough to tell what's what (plus, you don't want their individual scents to blend).

Once dried, store herbs in metal tins, lidded glass jars, plastic containers, or zip-seal plastic bags. Keep them in a cool spot away from moisture and sunlight to up their shelf life.

For more information on homegrown herbs, check out the individual herbs listed in Part 2 (page 49) for specific recommendations.

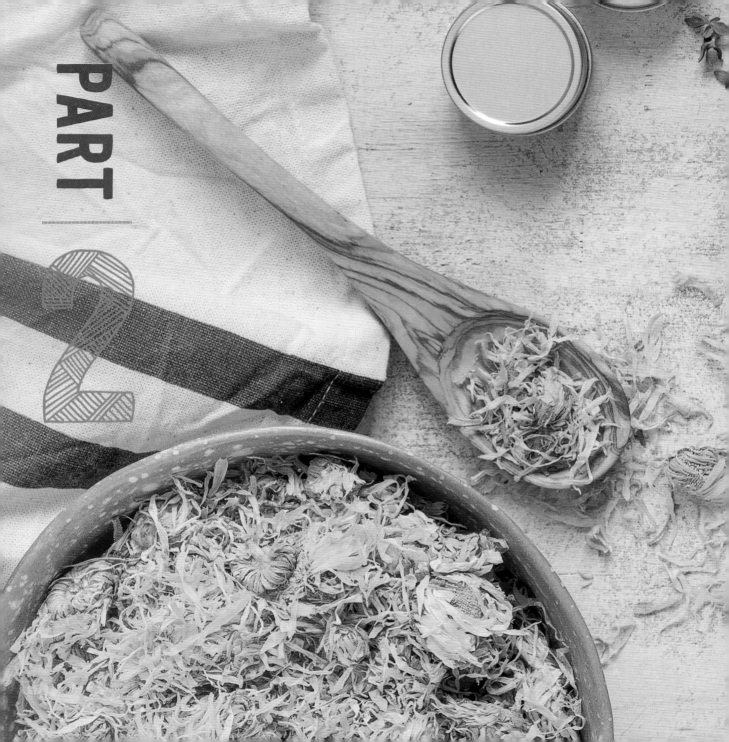

PART

2

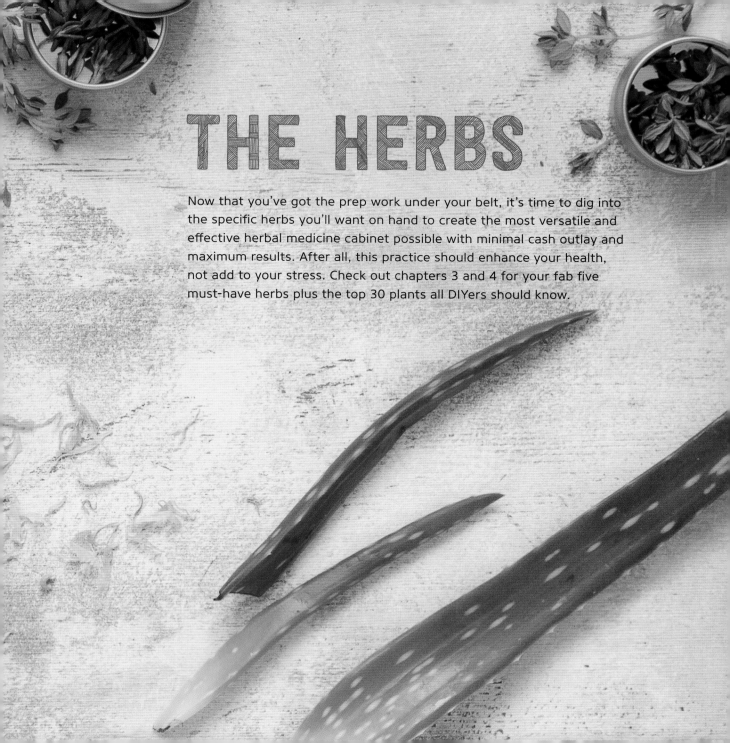

THE HERBS

Now that you've got the prep work under your belt, it's time to dig into the specific herbs you'll want on hand to create the most versatile and effective herbal medicine cabinet possible with minimal cash outlay and maximum results. After all, this practice should enhance your health, not add to your stress. Check out chapters 3 and 4 for your fab five must-have herbs plus the top 30 plants all DIYers should know.

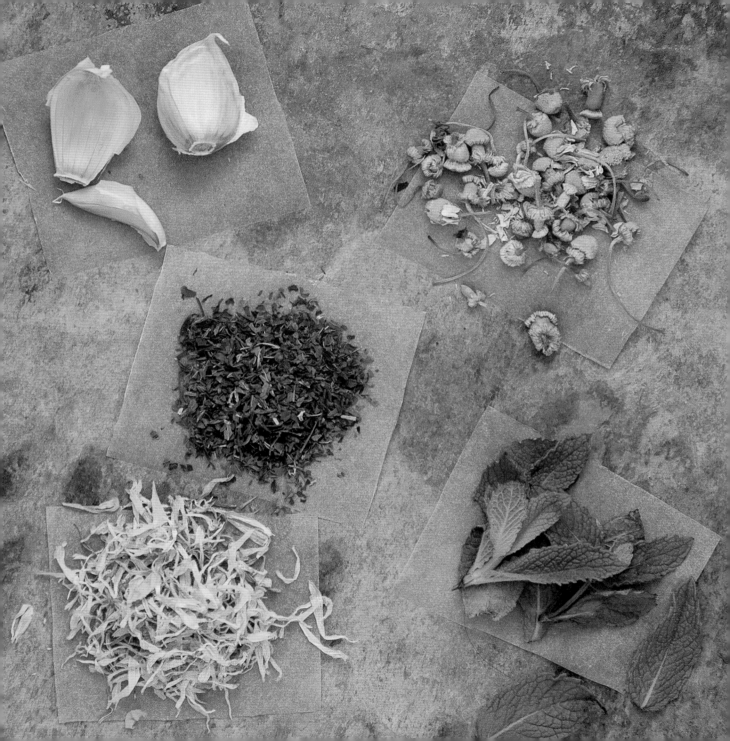

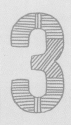

THE
FABULOUS FIVE

Your Must-Have Herbs

This section provides you with information about the herbs you'll want in your arsenal because they're highly versatile super healers. Stock up on these fab five and you'll instantly have access to a supply of healing options in a vast variety of preparations. Even better, you can use them before you need them because the powerhouses in this chapter work just as well in preventing ailments as they do in treating them.

CHAMOMILE (German and Roman)

MATRICARIA RECUTITA, CHAMAEMELUM NOBILE

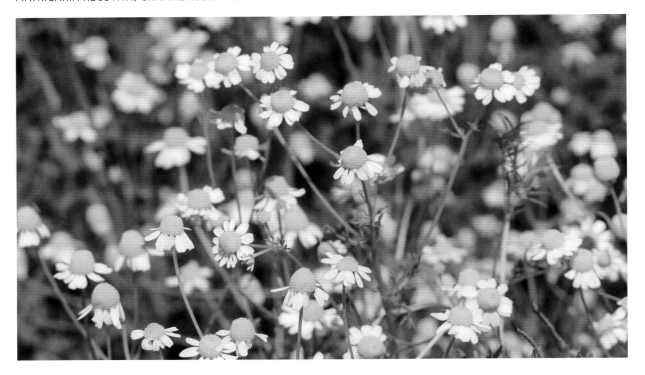

If there's one herb you can call a jack-of-all-trades, this one's it. Chamomile works wonders on a wide range of ailments, ranging from anxiety to upset stomach to pain relief. In terms of preparations, this easy-to-grow plant isn't just for teas anymore. Look for it in soothing skin tonics, healing lotions, and other beauty treatments with a purpose.

Did You Know?

In medieval times, chamomile was known as the "plant's physician" because wherever it was planted, flowers and herbs around it were healed and rejuvenated. Today, gardeners plant the herb to keep nearby flowers, vegetables, and plants healthy and disease free. In medical circles, chamomile is being studied and used around the world for a wide variety of conditions, each one remarkably different. For instance, it's been used to do everything from heal wounds and ease PMS, to treat Crohn's disease and lessen labor pains. Keep this "plant's physician" in your home so it's on hand whenever you need a healing remedy.

Why It's Essential

Twenty-six countries can't be wrong. Chamomile has been approved by more than two dozen nations to treat chronic and/or serious issues and ailments ranging from inflammation and infection to colic, muscle tension, and pain. Its active ingredients include azulene (known to be an antifever, anti-inflammatory substance) along with tannins, flavonoids, calcium, phosphorus, magnesium, salicylates, and bitter glycosides.

Herbal Power

MEDICINAL: Treats or prevents inflammatory conditions like arthritis, aches, pain; provides digestive support and nervous system support to calm, de-stress, and facilitate sleep; treats eczema, acne, psoriasis; heals chest colds, chicken pox, diaper rash, and slow-healing wounds.

COSMETIC: Used in facial teas, lotions, creams, and toners to treat blemishes, wrinkles, and redness; hair brightener and lightener.

Application Methods

- Apply as a cream, lotion, tincture, compress, or poultice
- Diffuse
- Drink as a tea or tonic
- Use in a bath

Precautions

Chamomile has a calming effect that can be sedating. Be aware of the effects before driving. Do not use if you're pregnant.

Other Names

Blue Chamomile
Wild Chamomile
Sweet Chamomile

Locating & Growing

- Easy-to-source seeds
- Plant in early spring, full sunlight, and rich soil

TREAT YOURSELF

TO SOME QUALITY ZZZS

Chamomile (and other calming flowers or herbs) can be sewn into bed pillows, bath pillows, eye masks, or sleep masks to enhance calm and promote a more restful slumber. Dream on!

ECHINACEA

ECHINACEA PURPUREA

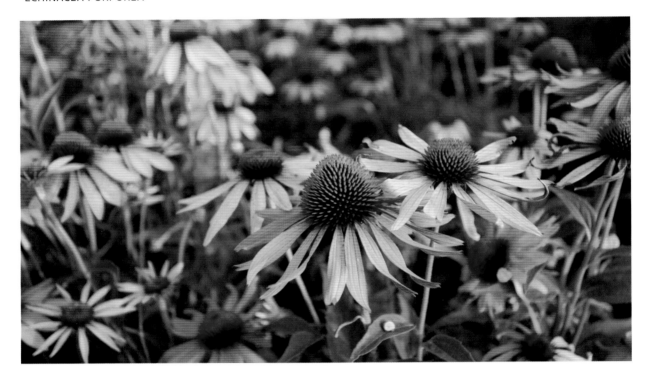

Grow this lifesaver in advance of cold and flu season and you'll be armed and ready to withstand viruses, bacteria, and anything else winter weather has to throw at you. This super herb is also a fantastic go-to for flawless, radiant skin, as well as treating skin issues or ailments like psoriasis, eczema, and bug bites. You'll readily find it as a whole herb, premade tablets, or essential oils, but since it's easy to grow, prep it in your kitchen to turn it into a tincture or tea.

Did You Know?

Native Americans looked to echinacea as their one-stop shop for healing. It was used to prevent and treat everything from colds and flu to snakebites, blood poisoning, and tooth infections. Early European explorers to the New World quickly caught on to the herb's magic and began using it to fight infections. Anthropologist Melvin Gilmore wrote that Plains Indians used echinacea as a "remedy for more ailments than any other plant."

Why It's Essential

More than just a cold fighter, this immune booster boasts a host of amazing nutrients and ingredients like caffeic acid, beta-carotene, vitamin C, linoleic acid, polysaccharides, echinacoside, tannins, and sesquiterpenes. Ask an herbalist and they'll likely tell you this is the single most significant immunity booster you can have in your plant arsenal.

Herbal Power

MEDICINAL: Boosts immunity by increasing T-cell production; repairs muscles and ligaments post-injury; heals cuts, bruises, burns, and wounds; eases pains and aches in muscles, throat, and head; features antifungal, antiviral, and antiseptic properties.

COSMETIC: Hydrates skin, lessens wrinkles, and boosts collagen.

Application Methods

- Apply as a cream, salve, lotion, splash, poultice, compress, or tincture
- Drink as a tea
- Use in a bath

Precautions

Allergic reactions to echinacea aren't uncommon. Stop using if you experience itchy eyes, ears, or throat or sinus congestion.

Other Names

Black Sampson Root
Kansas Snakeroot
Purple Coneflower

Locating & Growing

Echinacea grows just about anywhere under most conditions. In a perfect world, it loves full sun, warm weather, and rich soil, but it's known to survive harsh situations including drought.

A CLOSER LOOK

ECHINACEA CAN BE TOO MUCH OF A GOOD THING

Although this herb is an immunity-boosting powerhouse, it's not recommended to take high doses for more than a couple of weeks. Because it supercharges your immune system, over time it can stress the same system it works to bolster in the short-term. People with autoimmune diseases, in particular, should always consult a naturopath before undertaking an echinacea regimen.

GARLIC

ALLIUM SATIVUM

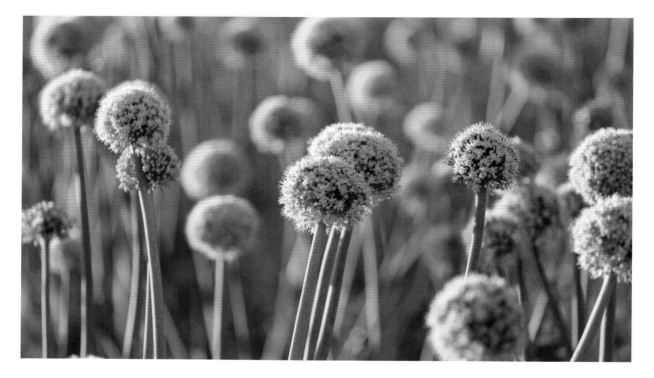

Many chefs would tell you if they could have just one ingredient in the kitchen, it would be garlic. Funnily enough, many herbalists say the same thing. Beyond being transformative in most culinary recipes, garlic is equally as life changing to your health. Add it to recipes throughout the year and eat raw or cooked to ward off disease, infection, colds, and flu. It's inexpensive, versatile, and aside from some minor breath issues, side effects are minimal to zilch.

Did You Know?

Not sure why, but it's said that ancient Greek and Roman brides carried bouquets of garlic and other herbs, rather than beautiful flower mixes, during their marriage ceremonies. Ancient Egyptians loved garlic, too. In fact, they fed it to the slaves who built the Great Pyramid, thinking it gave them super strength.

Why It's Essential

Check out this list of good-for-you ingredients, all packed into each clove: vitamins A, B, and C, magnesium, potassium, phosphorous, sulfur, germanium, selenium, alliin (the powerhouse that converts to allicin when broken or mashed), and essential oils. This cocktail of nutrients boasts an impressive success rate at fighting heart disease, cancers, and infection, while boosting immunity, warding off colds, and clearing blood of toxins. That's worth a little funky breath, right?

Herbal Power

MEDICINAL: Best for the heart and blood; it's antiseptic (internal and external) and bacteria-resistant; lowers cholesterol, lowers blood sugar levels, treats type 2 diabetes, boosts white blood cell count, and bolsters immunity; treats all types of cancer (rectal, stomach, prostate, breast, lung, colon); eases headaches and lowers stress.

COSMETIC: Some experts use garlic in combination with tea tree oil and egg whites in a purifying, cleansing, blemish-fighting face mask.

Application Methods

- Apply topically as a disinfectant
- Eat in foods, prepared raw, pickled, etc.

Precautions

Garlic can be irritating if used topically. Too much can cause heartburn or stomach issues.

Other Names

Ajo

Stinking Rose

Locating & Growing

Garlic thrives in full sunlight. Plant cloves points up in the autumn so you'll get your herbs by late summer, or plant in the spring to see bounty by late fall.

DOUBLE DUTY

SPLINTER REMOVAL

Yes, you read that right. Turns out, garlic has been used as a folk remedy for coaxing out painful slivers from under your skin—people still swear by it. Just duct tape or bandage a slice of garlic over the splinter before bed and wait until morning. Adios, splinter (and tweezers!).

PEPPERMINT

MENTHE PIPERITA

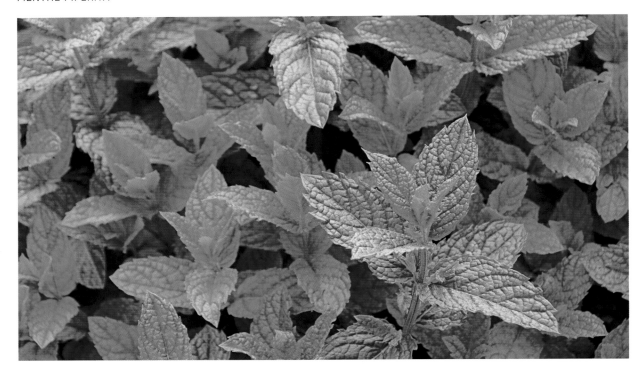

When you think of peppermint, it's likely that gum, candy, or chocolate comes to mind. But this brilliant herb does more than soothe a sweet tooth. This easy-to-grow plant is excellent to keep on hand not just for its ability to soothe an upset stomach, but also for its usefulness in relieving sinus, nasal, and chest congestion during cold and flu season. When applied externally, say in a poultice, compress, or herbal bath, it's fabulous for soothing sore or tired post-workout muscles and relieving pain from minor sprains and strains. Buy it in everything from seed to tea to essential oil.

Did You Know?

Ancient Romans were onto this herb long before modern medicine. They nibbled on peppermint to boost their smarts, smelled the herb to keep tempers quelled, and royals even stashed it in their pockets for on-the-go healing and energizing. Turns out, even the Romans were late to the game. Peppermint has been found in Egyptian tombs circa 1000 B.C., and before that, recorded in Chinese medicine.

Why It's Essential

Consider this multipurpose wonder an amazing pick-me-up for brains, emotions, moods, and spirit. It's energizing, restorative, rejuvenating, and cognitively stimulating. Experts say it boosts memory, cognition, and productivity. Unlike a midday shot of coffee, peppermint is naturally revitalizing so you don't have the post-sip crash. What's its secret? The herb is chock-full of flavonoids, phenolic acid, triterpines, calcium, magnesium, potassium, menthol, and menthone.

Herbal Power

MEDICINAL: Treats bee stings, headaches, toothaches, digestive distress, indigestion, burns, and bites; disinfects wounds; used as a mental stimulant and energizer.

COSMETIC: Cools, deodorizes, disinfects, and energizes skin, feet, mouth, and hair.

Application Methods

- Apply as a salve, tincture, compress, or poultice
- Drink as a tea
- Use in a bath
- Use in a room spray

Precautions

None documented; it's completely nontoxic

Other Names

Corn Mint
Lamb Mint

Locating & Growing

If you're looking at the USDA Plant Hardiness Zone Map, peppermint thrives in Zones 5 through 9. That said, it's wild at heart with survival instincts, so it can grow almost anywhere. Think full to partial sun and rich, moist soil if possible.

A CLOSER LOOK

PEPPERMINT IS A NATURAL DEODORANT

Add a few drops of peppermint essential oil to your body splash or foot scrub to leave skin with a fresh scent that lasts for hours. Or add a touch to your room spray or household cleaner so it disinfects and deodorizes while it stimulates your senses.

CALENDULA

CALENDULA OFFICINALIS

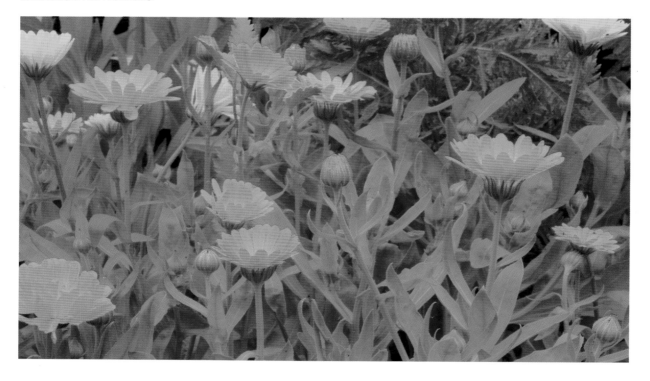

You'll love this soothing option for a wide range of medicinal uses. It makes a tasty healing tea for gastrointestinal or digestive issues, a brilliant first aid wash for wounds, an excellent healing balm for irritated or injured skin, a fabulously nourishing moisturizer, and a luscious all-natural soap. While it's commercially available as whole herb, infused oil, and tincture, it's also super easy to grow.

Did You Know?

Calendula can raise your A game at the dinner table. These amazing edible flowers brighten salads, soups, pastas, stews, omelets, and more with gourmet attitude, thanks to their brilliant yellow-orange shade. Their gorgeous blooms mask one of their best features: their heartiness. These flowers can withstand early frost and snow, while blooming year-round in temperate climates. For DIYers, this means calendula doesn't need your green thumb, it can take care of itself!

Why It's Essential

Thanks to a powerhouse roundup of active ingredients including bitters, volatile oils, resins, flavonoids, saponins, carotenoids, and mucilage, it's the go-to skin fixer for nearly all issues from dehydration to more serious concerns. Its non-toxicity makes it ideal for treating babies as well, especially as a go-to diaper rash cream. The herb is also valued for its effectiveness as an antiviral, anti-inflammatory, antimicrobial, and antiseptic. If that's not enough, try it as an aromatherapy tool to keep skin youthful, radiant, and flawless.

Herbal Power

MEDICINAL: Heals infections, bruises, sores, wounds, rashes, and other skin irritations and eruptions; reduces fever; treats ulcers, cramps, indigestion, and diarrhea; detoxes lymphatic systems and treats swollen glands; decongests lungs; energizes; supports heart, liver, gall bladder, and uterus.

COSMETIC: Soothes irritation, hydrates aging skin, tightens and firms sagginess.

Application Methods

- Apply as a poultice or salve
- Drink as a tea
- Use in a face cream or as a cleanser

Precautions

None documented; it's completely nontoxic

Other Names

Marigold
Hollygold

Locating & Growing

Plant in fall in your garden to bloom in early spring. Loves full sunshine, fertile soil, and occasional water but grows like a weed even if neglected.

A CLOSER LOOK

CALENDULA FIGHTS TO ERASE SCARS

A natural antiseptic and anti-inflammatory, calendula can help prevent, treat, and heal acne. But what about acne scars? Add a few drops of essential oil directly on the affected skin (or in your skin cream) and allow a few weeks for the redness and scarring to minimize as collagen production is stimulated.

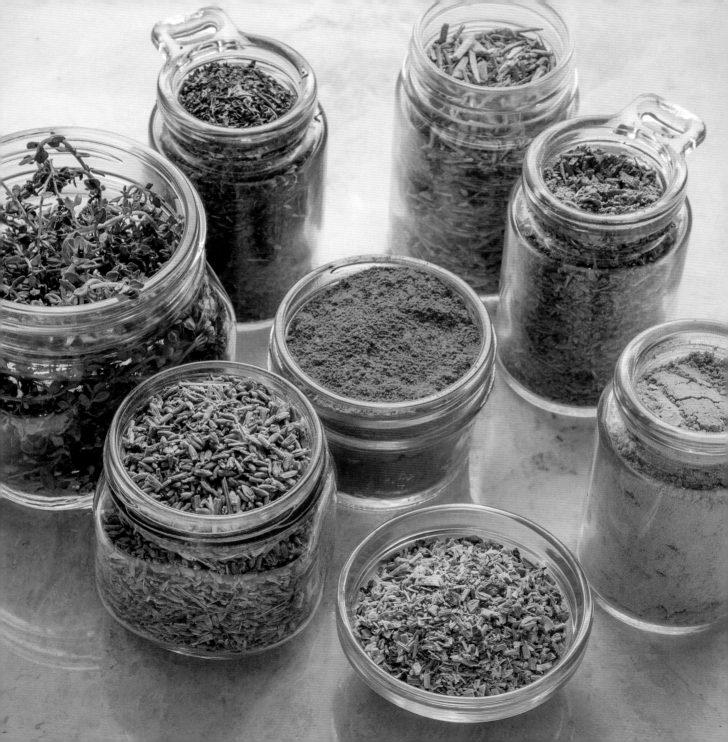

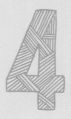

THE WORTHY THIRTY

Thirty Herbs
for Beauty and Overall Health

Modern society seems to be on an endless hunt for the wonder pill or proverbial Fountain of Youth that turns back the clock or renders us all ageless. The irony is that the greatest risk factors for disease and ailments—immunity destroyers like inflammation, stress, environmental pollutants, and more—can be eliminated or treated with items you've already got in your backyard, on your windowsill, or at the farmers' market. You already know the answer: herbs.

In this chapter you'll find profiles of the herbs you'll come back to again and again to deal with the side effects of living in a modern world. You'll get the scoop on where they're from, what they're good for, and why you need them in your life.

ALOE VERA

ALOE BARBADENSIS

Whether or not you're ready to go full-on with medicinal herbs, keeping an aloe vera plant in your house is a no-brainer. Besides being supremely simple to care for, it's useful to have on hand for on-demand first aid for burns, sunburns, scratches, or any other skin situation. Because it's loaded with tannins, vitamins E and B, fiber, selenium, polysaccharides, silicon, and aloin, you're just as likely to find it in an over-the-counter ointment as you are on the menu of a juice bar. For more serious issues, like arthritis pain, stomach issues, or inflammatory conditions, many herbalists keep a jar of store-bought aloe vera juice in their fridge to spike their morning cup of tea.

Did You Know?

Aloe is the ultimate beautifier, said to be a secret weapon in Cleopatra's skincare routine. Split open a leaf and use the gel straight up as a makeup remover, hair conditioner, or cuticle softener. There are brains behind all its beautifying power, too. Studies have shown it may be effectively used to treat diabetes and asthma.

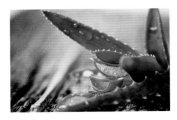

Herbal Power

MEDICINAL: Treats first-, second-, and third-degree burns and wounds; heals scars; reduces inflammation in eczema, skin ulcers, acne, rashes, stings, insect bites, and poison oak and ivy; soothes sunburns; eases intestinal disorders and inflammation-related pain.

COSMETIC: Balances pH levels in skin and blocks sunrays.

Application Methods

- Drink in juices, teas, tinctures, or smoothies
- Apply as an ointment/salve, face cream, lotion, bath, or splash
- Use as a tonic

Precautions

Aloe vera, if taken internally, can cause stomach cramping or distress. It also has laxative properties.

Other Names

Chinese Aloe
Indian Aloe
True Aloe
Barbados Aloe
Burn Aloe
First Aid Plant

Locating & Growing

Many herbalists consider this one of the easiest plants to grow and one that is almost impossible to harm. It's happy indoors or outdoors, in sunlight or shade, in rain or dry conditions. If you can manage to give it a touch of UV rays and a spritz of water every now and then, it's golden.

ARNICA

ARNICA MONTANA

Plant some arnica in your garden and you'll have this perennial for at least two springs. You'll recognize this medicinal beauty because of its bright yellow, daisy-like appearance and round, hairy stems. Although its active ingredients are primarily known to be analgesic and anti-inflammatory, some herbalists use it as an antibiotic, particularly for topical skin conditions.

Did You Know?

Arnica has been revered since the 1600s for its pain-relieving prowess. German philosopher Goethe is rumored to have smoked its leaves and drank its tea to relieve chest pain. Recently, numerous studies have concluded that the herb is effective for relieving muscle pain due to strenuous exercise. In fact, a 2003 study published in *Homeopathy* showed it worked better than a placebo for treating muscle soreness on runners who just completed a 26.2-mile marathon.

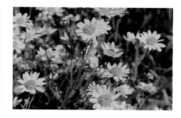

Herbal Power

MEDICINAL: Reduces muscle and joint pain and related swelling; treats osteoarthritis, bruises, acne, sore throats, and insect bites; nourishes chapped lips; eases symptoms of stroke.

COSMETIC: Treats dandruff, nourishes hair, promotes hair growth, and sweetly scents cosmetics and fragrances.

Application Methods

- Drink as a highly diluted tea or tincture
- Use externally in gels, salves, ointments, oils, poultices, sprays, hair tonics, lip balms, and other topical preparations

Precautions

Arnica is generally considered toxic in amounts greater than what you'd find in food or cosmetics. In fact, the amount you find in homeopathic or herbal remedies is generally so diluted it's considered safe. Don't use on broken skin, before or after surgery (it increases circulation), or if you have digestive conditions. It's considered unsafe to inhale or use as aromatherapy.

Other Names

Leopard's Bane
Mountain Tobacco
Wolf's Bane

Locating & Growing

Like many herbs, arnica is hardy and works well in nearly all temperate climates. A native of the mountainous European and Asian regions, you'll likely find arnica in northern areas of the United States and at higher altitudes. In fact, it's not unlikely to find it on your next hiking trip in the Rockies, as high as 8,000 feet according to some reports.

BLACK COHOSH

ACTAEA RACEMOSA

Black cohosh will become your best friend if you experience painful or uncomfortable menopausal or PMS symptoms. The combination of its active ingredients—tannins, resins, fatty acids, 27-deoxyactein, isoflavones, triterpene glycosides, and formononetin—simulates the hormone estrogen and has been clinically proven to ease fever, cramps, bloating, mood swings, depression, and more.

Did You Know?

North American Indians used black cohosh to treat gynecological conditions, kidney problems, malaria, snake bites, coughs, and colds. Later it was used as a home remedy, as a diuretic, and to trigger menstruation. Herbalists have since primarily focused its use on women's pain related to the uterus, ovaries, infertility, and labor, while it's also used in alternative remedies for neurological and lung disorders.

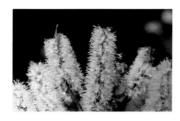

Herbal Power

MEDICINAL: Treats menopause symptoms, such as hot flashes, insomnia, and related depression; suppresses appetite and stimulates metabolism.

COSMETIC: Treats acne.

Application Methods

- Drink as a tea
- Use in tinctures or extracts

Precautions

Researchers recommend not taking black cohosh if you're breastfeeding, pregnant, diagnosed with breast cancer, or have hormone-sensitive issues that would be triggered by the herb, which simulates estrogen in the body. If you take the herb internally, take a break after one year. Also stop if you're experiencing side effects like upset stomach, headaches, cramps, weight gain, spotting, or bleeding between menstrual periods.

Other Names

Baneberry
Black Snakeroot
Bugbane
Phytoestrogen
Rattlesnake Root
Rattleweed
Sheng Ma
Snakeroot
Squaw Root

Locating & Growing

Black cohosh likes to be left in the dark, preferring shade or partial shade over sunlight. It thrives in moist, organic dirt and must experience a complete cycle of warm to cold to warm again before the seeds will germinate. Ensure success by planting mature seeds in fall so it experiences the cycle and up your odds of growing during its first spring.

BURDOCK

If you've had Japanese takeout recently, chances are you've had burdock root. Not only does it taste fantastic, it's also loaded with anti-inflammatory, antioxidant, anticancer, antibacterial, and other healing attributes. New studies have even shown that it may be a prebiotic, which supports the growth of beneficial bacteria in your intestines and keeps you healthy, even in cold and flu season. If you make it as a side dish at home, gourmets and herbalists will tell you two things: Leave on the skin—it's got massive nutrients— and soak the roots for 15 to 20 minutes prior to broiling, boiling, or sautéing to lose its bitter, muddy notes. Don't worry, it's tastier than it sounds.

Did You Know?

Most recently, burdock had its 15 minutes of fame in the '90s with the explosion of Velcro. Its inventor, George de Mestral, created the fabric fastening device in 1948 after going on a hiking trip with his dog and finding burdock burrs stuck on his clothing and his best friend's fur.

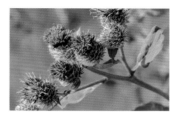

Herbal Power

MEDICINAL: Treats a variety of skin issues from psoriasis and eczema to acne and rashes; supports the liver, heart, and related conditions like hypertension, poor digestion, heart disease, and gas.

COSMETIC: Treats dry, irritated scalps.

Application Methods

- Apply as a poultice, compress, or tincture
- Drink as a tea
- Eat in food

Precautions

No toxicity levels reported. Herbalists consider this among the safest plants to grow and use.

Other Names

Beggar's Buttons
Burr Seed
Cocklebur
Fox's Clote
Niu Bang Zi
Personata
Thorny Burr

Locating & Growing

Burdock is one of those aggressive, impossible-to-destroy weeds that you've probably tried to destroy if you've got a garden. That is, before you learned about its incredible healing potential. A true survivor, this herb grows on just about any soil from dry to rocky to moist, survives freezes and droughts, and doesn't have a preference about sunlight.

CAYENNE

CAPSICUM ANNUUM

If you can't take the heat, you might want to up your tolerance. Cayenne is more than just a spicy flower, it's a health superfood. Chock-full of vitamins A, B₆, and C, manganese, potassium, beta-carotene, capsaicin, carotenoids, flavonoids, and oils, it acts as a natural anti-allergen, antifungal, anti-irritant, and anti-inflammatory. This amazing little spice does in your body what it does to your mouth—makes things hot fast. How does that translate into health? It speeds healing, quickens circulation, ups metabolism, boosts immunity, and spurs hair growth. It's like a shot of adrenaline right to your health.

Did You Know?

Capsaicin, the ingredient that dials up the heat in the pepper, has been widely studied for its healing properties. Scientists have looked at more than 300 studies of its effects on metabolism and shown that it does speed weight loss and temper appetite.

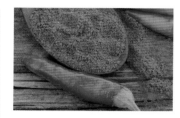

Herbal Power

MEDICINAL: Eases sore throat, muscle aches, back pain, migraines, and painful joints; fights colds; aids digestion and circulation; boosts immunity; treats skin conditions like psoriasis; cures ear infections; speeds weight loss by increasing metabolism.

COSMETIC: Triggers hair growth; decreases acne; reduces wrinkles; revitalizes tired and aging eye areas.

Application Methods

- Eat in food
- Apply as a salve, massage oil, or tincture

Precautions

This is a very spicy herb and should be handled with care especially for those with sensitive skin. Wear gloves and/or wash hands thoroughly after use to avoid getting it into your eyes. Also, beware that large doses can upset your stomach. Less is more with cayenne.

Other Names

African Pepper
Bird Pepper
Capsaicin
Chili
Red Pepper
Tabasco Pepper

Locating & Growing

As you'd expect, cayenne prefers things hot. It's a summertime herb that thrives in full sun, warm weather, and rich soil.

Clove is a highly nutrient-dense spice whose active ingredient, eugenol, has been studied widely. Packed with manganese, iron, magnesium, calcium, vitamin K, and fiber, this wonder flower bud is revered for its anti-inflammatory, antiviral, antibacterial, and analgesic properties. Although studies are inconclusive, it's being used to supplement modern cancer care and treatments as well as other conditions like hepatitis with positive results.

Did You Know?

Since the eighth century, cloves were a major part of European and Asian commerce. In fact, wars have been fought over the spice. Today, Indonesia accounts for half of the world's consumption of cloves.

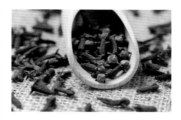

Herbal Power

MEDICINAL: Treats cuts, wounds, burns, throat issues, earaches, nausea, diabetes, headaches, sore gums, bites, stings, and tooth decay; boosts immunity, libido, and brain function; battles stress, fatigue, depression, anxiety, memory loss, insomnia, and premature ejaculation; stimulates circulation.

COSMETIC: Treats bad breath, acne, wrinkles, sagging skin, and dryness.

Application Methods

- Apply as an oil, ointment, poultice, skincare cream, or fragrance
- Drink as a tea
- Eat in food
- Use for aromatherapy or in soap

Precautions

Clove is considered safe when taken in amounts typically found in foods; however, no studies have been done taking the herb for medicinal use in the long term. Children, pregnant women, and breastfeeding women should avoid medicinal doses because it's untested. The active ingredient in clove, eugenol, slows blood clotting, so avoid ingesting clove post-surgery or if you're taking blood thinners.

Other Names

Clove Flower
Clove Leaf
Clove Oil
Ding Xiang
Eugenia Aromatica
Oil of Clove

Locating & Growing

Cloves are the flowering buds of perennial clove trees. They grow easily in wet, tropical areas or rich, red soil. Their ideal conditions are partial shade and rainfall. It takes 20 years for this plant to grow clove buds.

COMFREY

SYMPHYTUM

Comfrey features an impressive cocktail of skin-healing compounds including allantoin, tannins, rosmarinic acid, saponins, calcium, potassium, magnesium, chromium, and vitamins A, B, and C. Its leaves and stems are antioxidant, anti-inflammatory, antibacterial, and age-defying when added to skincare.

Did You Know?

This herb was a secret beauty ingredient with ancient civilizations for its skin-healing, anti-aging, and youth-promoting effects. It moisturizes, triggers skin cell turnover, brightens, protects from bacteria, inflammation, and redness, and nourishes skin layers. You'll find it in beauty products like scrubs, masks, night creams, and blemish fighters. In the Middle Ages, it was renowned for treating broken bones, although modern scientists have yet to confirm that this particular remedy works.

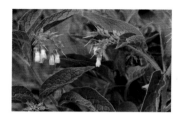

Herbal Power

MEDICINAL: Treats back pain, osteoarthritis, sprains, bruises, wounds, sore throat, joint pain, chest pain, and inflammation.

COSMETIC: Renews and rejuvenates skin, spurs cell turnover, fights wrinkles, and protects from UV damage.

Application Methods

- Apply as an ointment, oil, salve, poultice, compress, facial scrub, or anti-aging cream
- Use as an extract

Precautions

It's not recommended to take comfrey by mouth due to its pyrrolizidine alkaloids, which can cause lung disease, cancer, and liver damage. It's best used topically on unbroken skin for periods less than 10 days. Avoid if pregnant or breastfeeding.

Other Names

Ass Ear
Black Root
Blackwort
Gum Plant
Healing Herb
Knitback
Slippery Root
Wallwort

Locating & Growing

You'll love comfrey in your garden because its vivid blue and purple flowers look fantastic, it's easy to grow, and it thrives under the shade of other trees and plants. Only downside is that if you ever want to get rid of it, good luck. Its roots are brittle and breakable, and sprout new plants readily and easily.

EUCALYPTUS

EUCALYPTUS GLOBULUS

Eucalyptus gets its name from its powerful active ingredient eucalyptol, which makes up about 70 percent of its compounds. It has effective anti-inflammatory, analgesic, antiseptic, antiviral, decongestant, and disinfectant properties. Its woodsy oils make a potent aromatherapy tool for balancing and stimulating the mind, body, and emotions, as well as healing viral infections and respiratory conditions. Using the herb for steam inhalation is also fantastic for clearing out the lungs, opening nasal passages, and treating sinuses.

Did You Know?

With more than 300 species and 700 different varieties, eucalyptus has been a favorite among healers for centuries. Aborigines used it to disinfect wounds, lessen pain, and drive down fevers. The tree has also been a mainstay of Traditional Chinese Medicine. Taken at the onset of colds, fever, flu, sinusitis, bronchitis, or other infections, it's said to speed healing and shorten sickness.

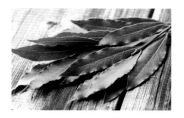

Herbal Power

MEDICINAL: Treats infections, fever, osteoarthritis, joint pain, upset stomach, coughs, liver and gallbladder issues, ulcers, burns, respiratory problems, asthma, wounds, ulcers, and depression; repels insects.

COSMETIC: Fights acne.

Application Methods

- Apply as an ointment, gel, salve, compress, oil, or splash

Precautions

Eucalyptus should be diluted before applying topically to skin. If you've got diabetes, note that eucalyptus has been shown in studies to lower blood sugar.

Other Names

Blue Gum
Fever Tree
Gully Gum
Red Gum
Stringy Bark Tree

Locating & Growing

Growing eucalyptus indoors is easy and quite common. It needs full sunlight and well-drained soil. Keep temps between 50 and 75 degrees Fahrenheit. If you're planting outdoors, heads up that this tree won't reach its full height potential unless you live in a warm climate.

GERANIUM

PELARGONIUM

Geranium's mother country is South Africa but it has been used around the world for centuries to fight infections, colds, wounds, and more. A powerful astringent, it is known for opening, cleaning, and shrinking the size of your pores (a beauty must-have for youthful skin). You'll find it in tonics, toners, skin creams, serums, and moisturizers. Also a mood booster, add it to a diffuser on your office desk or near your bath to heighten spirits and combat stress. Herbalists (along with centuries of anecdotal evidence from healers and doctors) say it's worth adding to your arsenal of remedies for its anti-inflammatory, antiseptic, and antibacterial properties.

Did You Know?

Early settlers to North America used it for stomach ailments like diarrhea, cramps, and gastric ulcers as well as sexually transmitted diseases (STDs) and killing lice. A known infection fighter, geranium is used to ease heavy menstrual flow, and in remedies for vaginal infections, toothaches, and even severe issues like typhoid fever.

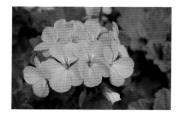

Herbal Power

MEDICINAL: Treats digestive conditions, irritable bowel syndrome (IBS), canker sores, gum disease, vaginal discharge, hemorrhoids, wounds, and bleeding; balances hormones, menstruation, and moods; detoxifies system.

COSMETIC: Works as an astringent.

Application Methods

- Apply as a tincture or oil
- Drink as a tea
- Eat in food
- Use in aromatherapy
- Use as an astringent in toners, splashes, tonics, creams, or shampoos

Precautions

Spotted geranium is generally considered safe with no known risks or side effects reported.

Other Names

Cranesbill
Spotted Cranesbill
Wild Geranium
Wood Geranium

Locating & Growing

Geraniums are fairly easy to grow, able to withstand a variety of harsh conditions like drought or heat. Their perfect situation is full sunlight, warm temps, and a covered location, making it ideal for a windowsill indoors.

As an all-around cure-all and immunity booster (thanks to healing ketones like gingerol), ginger rivals its culinary counterpart, garlic, in effectiveness in treating a variety of conditions. You've likely already been enjoying its medicinal benefits if you're a fan of Thai, Indian, or Chinese cooking. Like garlic, you can get enormous healing benefits by incorporating the herb into your culinary routine more regularly.

Did You Know?

No matter how you cut it (pickle it, crystallize it, or put it in a tea bag), ginger's medicinal properties made it one of the most coveted and prized plants throughout the world and over the rise and fall of many empires. In the thirteenth and fourteenth centuries, it's believed that a pound of ginger would set you back the price of one sheep. Despite its well-documented use, no one is sure of the plant's origins.

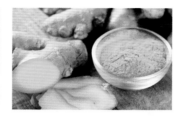

Herbal Power

MEDICINAL: Treats inflammation, swollen joints, damaged cartilage, arthritis pain, muscle pain, PMS symptoms, high cholesterol, colds, flu, poor circulation, nausea, congestion, sore throat, motion sickness, and chemotherapy side effects; supports reproductive issues with men.

COSMETIC: Combats aging; improves skin tone; calms irritation; smooths skin surface; adds warmth and spicy fragrance to skincare products.

Application Methods

- Drink as a tea
- Use in oils
- Eat in foods
- Use as a poultice, compress, mask, scrub, body and face cream, or serum

Precautions

Ginger is considered safe and nontoxic.

Other Names

African Ginger
Ginger Root
Indian Ginger
Jamaica Ginger
Jiang
Shen Jiang

Locating & Growing

Ginger thrives in conditions similar to its native Asia: hot, sunny, humid, moist soil. If you care for ginger indoors, it will likely go dormant during the winter months.

GINSENG

PANAX GINSENG

While ginseng has been a major component of Traditional Chinese Medicine for thousands of years, it's only recently come into vogue in the United States, having been studied for a variety of diseases and conditions ranging from mild to severe. The herb is a major force in strengthening immunity and treating digestive, heart, and nervous system issues, as well as a powerful addition to an anti-aging beauty regimen.

Did You Know?

The English word *ginseng* derives from the Chinese term that means "person" and "plant root." The root's characteristic forked shape resembles the legs of a person. The botanical/genus name, *panax*, means "all-heal" in Greek, sharing the same origin as *panacea*. Several studies show a link between ginseng and lower cancer risk, according to the American Cancer Society.

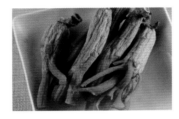

Herbal Power

MEDICINAL: Treats flu, colds, diabetes, depression, anxiety, heart issues, digestive problems, anemia, nerve pain, and fatigue; stops hardening of arteries; triggers metabolism; stabilizes blood sugar, mood, mental health, and insulin levels; lowers cholesterol; boosts immunity; heals erectile dysfunction.

COSMETIC: Stimulates cell turnover and hair growth; evens skin tone, smooths texture, and tones; treats under-eye wrinkles and dark circles.

Application Methods

- Eat in foods
- Use in powders or teas

Precautions

While it's considered safe and nontoxic, some people experience side effects including nausea, fatigue, dizziness, headaches, rapid heartbeat, and hypertension.

Other Names

American Ginseng
Canadian Ginseng
Panax Quinquefolia
Red Berry
Ren Shen
Shang
Shi Yang Seng

Locating & Growing

Got 5 to 10 years? That's how long it takes ginseng to reach maturity before you harvest. Your best bet is to buy older roots—say three to four years old—and plant them in spring. They prefer shade beneath other tree canopies and moist, well-drained soils.

GOLDENSEAL

HYDRASTIS CANADENSIS

A native to North America, goldenseal was commonly used by Native American tribes to protect against just about everything. Its main active ingredients—berberine and beta-hydrastine—have massive antimicrobial and astringent benefits, and it's also a powerful antibacterial, antiviral, and decongestant. Normally found in the wild, the huge market demand on this wonder herb has put its supplies in danger, so beware of any goldenseal product labels that don't say "organically cultivated."

Did You Know?

Perhaps you've heard through the grapevine about one of goldenseal's most popular uses—to produce a false negative when urine is tested for illegal drugs, from marijuana to cocaine. But according to the University of Maryland Medical Center, there's no hard evidence showing that goldenseal actually works for this purpose. As WebMD notes, the idea that goldenseal could alter the results first came up in a novel, and not a medical study.

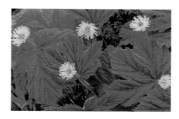

Herbal Power

MEDICINAL: Treats skin infections, bronchitis, digestive problems, colds, flu, reproductive issues, vaginal conditions, eye infections, mouth issues, eczema, psoriasis, acne, wounds, and ulcers; protects the liver; fights cancer; lowers cholesterol; and boosts immunity.

COSMETIC: Fights acne and soothes skin irritation.

Application Methods

- Drink as a tea
- Apply as a tincture, salve, ointment, oil, poultice, or compress

Precautions

Herbalists recommend taking breaks when consuming the herb internally—three weeks on, one week off—to stop irritation in the mucous membranes.

Other Names

Chinese Goldenseal
Eye Balm
Eye Root
Goldenroot
Hydraste
Indian Plant
Indian Turmeric

Locating & Growing

Consider goldenseal to be another high-maintenance herb with very particular needs to achieve optimal growth. Because it's a native of forested areas in Canada and the eastern United States, it thrives in similar climates and conditions: three-quarters shade and beneath a large tree. Soil should be humus-rich. That said, even if you get its gardening demands correct, you still have a three-year wait for a harvest.

HOPS

HUMULUS

Hops are the female flower of the hops plant. If you've ever done a pub crawl, you're aware of one of the biggest medicinal benefits of hops: its sedative effects. Over the years the herb has been shown to be effective at triggering weight loss, treating menstrual symptoms, soothing anxiety, and balancing moods. And not just when it's brewed and packed in a beer can. It's used today in a variety of preparations from teas to anti-aging skincare.

Did You Know?

Thanks to its popularity in home brewing (versus home healing), it's estimated that in pre-war times, nearly three-quarters of hops production was DIY at-home blends. (There's no record on how much was drunk out of a mug versus put into a medicine tincture.)

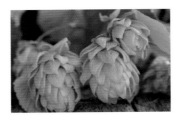

Herbal Power

MEDICINAL: Treats anxiety, insomnia, ADHD, mood issues (like irritability, tension, and excitability), stomach cramps, intestinal issues, nerve pain, and indigestion; balances hormones; promotes sleep; detoxes liver.

COSMETIC: Treats overworked, dry, or irritated skin; heals and moisturizes skin.

Application Methods

- Apply as a cream, lotion, or toner
- Drink as a tea or tonic
- Use in a bath
- Use as a tincture

Precautions

Hops are considered safe and nontoxic. However, some people should take care when using because they can make depression worse. They also simulate estrogen so avoid if you've been diagnosed with breast cancer. Hops may also interact with anesthesia, causing the patient to experience heightened effects. Hops are known to be harmful to dogs.

Other Names

Humulus Lupulus
Lupuli Strobulus
Pi Jiu Hua

Locating & Growing

If you've got rich, deep soil with southern exposure, you're in business. Keep the plant well watered and give it a place to climb.

HYSSOP

Hyssop gets its star power in the herbal medicine world from its properties as an antiseptic, cough reliever, expectorant, and for its aromatic qualities. It's revered by gourmet chefs for the flavor-enhancing kick it gives to soups, stews, salads, and sauces.

Did You Know?

This herb was another favorite of the Greeks, namely Hippocrates, Galen, and Dioscorides. In their times, the herb was readily recommended for a variety of issues—most popularly as a decongestant, disinfectant, and sedative. Today, its antiviral benefits are sought by those who have muscle tension, neck pain, stress, or throat complications due to overworking their voices. Actors, public speakers, singers, politicians, teachers, and others might find hyssop's performance quite useful. Add its essential oils to a carrier oil and it makes a fantastic massage or bath oil, or combine with almost any oil for a nourishing, antibacterial facial treatment.

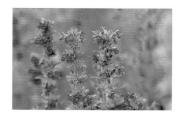

Herbal Power

MEDICINAL: Treats liver and gallbladder problems, intestinal cramps, colic, gas, asthma, sore throat, colds, flu, respiratory issues, urinary tract infections, HIV/AIDS, menstrual cramps, burns, bruises, frostbite, and skin irritations; triggers appetite.

COSMETIC: Adds a camphor scent to fragrances and cleaners.

Application Methods

- Eat in foods
- Use in soaps, cleaners, cosmetics, aromatherapy, oils, baths, and mouthwash

Precautions

Hyssop is known to be safe in low doses with a few exceptions. Because it's packed with ketones, avoid if pregnant because the herb may cause uterine cramps or trigger the onset of menstruation. If you're prone to seizures, avoid taking this herb because it may spur their onset and/or heighten them.

Other Names

Herbe de Joseph
Hiope
Hysope
Jufa
Ysop

Locating & Growing

A perennial shrub in the mint family, hyssop likes it hot, hot, hot. Look for the herb in dry, rocky conditions in full sunlight. If you want this herb in your own garden, start by propagating seeds indoors about eight weeks prior to your first frost. It's just as easy, however, to find them already grown in your local nursery or farmers' market or online.

LAVENDER

LAVANDULA ANGUSTIFOLIA

Lavender is no one-hit wonder. A powerfully effective and well-studied anti-inflammatory, anti-allergen, antibacterial, antispasmodic, and antiseptic, its uses range from anti-aging skincare to kitchen surface cleaner. In fact, it's one of the few essential oils that herbalists recommend applying directly to the skin for healing cuts, scrapes, wounds, and bruises with zero side effects.

Did You Know?

In Roman times, a pound of lavender flowers would set you back about a month's wages if you were a farm worker. The Greeks discovered early on that crushed and properly treated lavender would release a relaxing fume when burned. Later it was used for smoking, mummifying, and perfuming. French chemist René-Maurice Gattefossé, who coined the term *aromatherapy*, suffered terrible burns after a lab explosion. In a last-ditch effort at healing, he rubbed his burns with lavender essential oils, which sped healing and left his skin virtually scar-free.

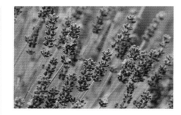

Herbal Power

MEDICINAL: Treats colds, flu, staph, strep, skin infections, nail infections, indigestion, muscle spasms, IBS, Crohn's disease, stress, fatigue, tension, depression, sadness, insomnia, and yeast infections; heals burns, wounds, cuts, and bruises.

COSMETIC: Erases wrinkles; banishes acne, psoriasis, eczema, and other skin conditions; triggers cell turnover; treats oiliness; tones, smooths, and evens skin.

Application Methods

- Apply as a balm, salve, ointment, or compress
- Drink as a tea or tonic
- Use in baths, cleaning solutions, sachets, aromatherapy, soaps, powders, or candles

Precautions

Lavender is considered safe and nontoxic, however, pregnant women should avoid taking large doses internally.

Other Names

English Lavender
French Lavender
Garden Lavender
Lavande
Lavandula
Spike Lavender
True Lavender

Locating & Growing

A perennial, lavender is a hardy plant able to grow just about anywhere. In fact, you've probably seen it growing in meadows, near roadsides, and in lush, wooded areas. While its natural habitat makes it suitable for Zones 5 to 8, give this herb some sun, warmth, and moist, well-drained soil, and it's a happy camper.

LEMON BALM

MELISSA OFFICINALIS

Lemon balm smells so strikingly fantastic, you'll almost forget it's a highly potent anti-inflammatory, antiviral, antispasmodic, and antibacterial agent. It's a natural remedy for digestive disorders, mood conditions, viruses like herpes and shingles, and feelings of grief, depression, and sadness. While most people put this luscious herb in the garden for its fragrant aroma, they soon find the effects on their mood to be transformative and uplifting. A recent study has shown that the herb's antioxidant and polyphenol profile improves memory, clarity, and focus, and may be able to combat Alzheimer's disease and cell oxidation.

Did You Know?

Lemon balm was used during the Middle Ages throughout Europe by Greeks and Romans for everything from dressing sword wounds to reversing baldness to treating fainting. Thought to be "an elixir of life" at one point, doctors weren't too far off, given what's known today by scientists.

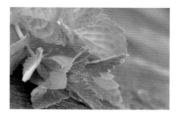

Herbal Power

MEDICINAL: Treats colic, insomnia, stress, worry, anxiety, fatigue, grief, depression, SAD (Seasonal Affective Disorder), ADD, ADHD, stomach issues, mood imbalances, and muscle spasms.

COSMETIC: Heals acne and sunburn; protects against UV rays; increases circulation and radiance; calms, soothes, and fights inflammation; evens skin tone; enhances fragrance in perfumes, candles, and body products.

Application Methods

- Apply as a tincture
- Drink as a tea or tonic
- Eat in foods
- Use in a bath, aromatherapy, candle, soap, or as a cleaner

Precautions

Lemon balm is considered safe with the exception of those with hypothyroidism or low thyroid activity. Consult your doctor before taking if you've got thyroid issues.

Other Names

Cure-All
Dropsy Plant
Honey Plant
Sweet Balm
Sweet Mary

Locating & Growing

The key to getting lemon balm growing is to make sure you get a couple of plants started and it will self sow. Ideal for Zones 4 to 9, it prefers moist soil and full to partial sun.

LICORICE

GLYCYRRHIZA GLABRA

The real herb (rather than the candy) is naturally sweet—50 times sweeter than sugar, in fact—and full of healing compounds. Even more shocking, the ingredient that makes licorice so sweet (glycyrrhizic acid) is one of the root's secret weapons thanks to its anti-inflammatory, antiviral, and anti-arthritic benefits that mimic hydrocortisone and corticosteroids in the body.

Did You Know?

While much of licorice's benefits are still considered lore—although the herb has been used extensively throughout Europe and Asia for centuries—an injectable form of the plant was shown in clinical trial to effectively fight hepatitis C.

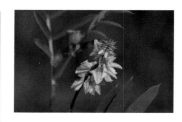

Herbal Power

MEDICINAL: Soothes inflammation, irritation, and pain; fights infections like shingles, herpes, colds, and bronchitis; treats ulcers, stomach cramps, prostate cancer, eczema, sore throat, constipation, adrenal fatigue, laryngitis, and throat stress and infections.

COSMETIC: Soothes rosacea, triggers cell turnover, rejuvenates skin, protects cell DNA, prevents breakouts, and smooths texture.

Application Methods

- Apply as an ointment, salve, or skin cream
- Drink as a tea or tonic
- Eat in food

Precautions

The active ingredient glycyrrhizic acid can stress the kidneys and heart due to its potential to deplete potassium and retain sodium. Check with your doctor before using if you've got high blood pressure, water retention, or heart palpitations.

Other Names

Chinese Licorice
Gan Zao
Licorice Root
Phytoestrogen
Sweet Root

Locating & Growing

Herbalists say that licorice falls into the category of "Mediterranean plant." In other words, it likes full sun, high heat, and sandy to partially sandy soil. If you're raising this herb indoors, know that if you take it from seed to harvest, you'll need about three years before it's ready to use medicinally.

MULLEIN

An expectorant and antispasmodic, this incredible plant does wonders for lung health both as a preventive and as a treatment. While some researchers have questioned its effectiveness as an antibacterial, others at Clemson University found mullein to successfully fight bacteria like *Staphylococcus aureus, Staphylococcus epidermis, E. coli,* and pneumonia.

Did You Know?

Another European plant originally thought to ward off evil spirits, this particular herb was considered one of the 23 most powerful healers in medieval Jewish medicine. Its leaves have since been used to start fires while the smoke is inhaled to treat lung issues like congestion, asthma, and cough.

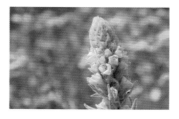

Herbal Power

MEDICINAL: Treats bronchial and respiratory conditions like cough, colds, chest colds, sore throats, and allergies; relieves pain; fights infections; heals skin conditions and ear infections.

COSMETIC: Detoxifies skin.

Application Methods

- Apply as a salve, poultice, compress, or oil
- Drink as a tea or tonic
- Use in a bath

Precautions

It's known to be safe and nontoxic. Some people are sensitive to the leaf's tiny hairs when applied topically.

Other Names

American Mullein
Beggar's Blanket
Blanket Herb
Candleflower
Lungwort
Torch Weed
Velvet Plant
Wild Ice Leaf
Woolly Mullein

Locating & Growing

Mullein, a biennial, makes a great addition to any garden—it's attractive and lures in both birds and bees. While it thrives in Zones 3 to 8, it's pretty happy anywhere you plant it. If you're into nature walks or outdoor exploration, you've probably seen it growing in the wild in fields, by streams, in woods, or next to highways. (It's easy to spot, given its skinny, stalk-like stem and seven-foot stature.)

PASSIONFLOWER

PASSIFLORA

Meet Mother Nature's wonder flower whose compounds have calming, sleep-inducing effects. In fact, the plant was once FDA-approved as an over-the-counter remedy for insomnia, but due to lack of evidence about its safety and effectiveness, it was pulled from the market in 1978. If you want those effects now, simply brew some passionflower tea, stash some of the fresh herbs under your pillow, and let the Zzzs begin.

Did You Know?

Passionflower may also be Mother Nature's remedy for psychological and brain issues related to anxiety, mood, stress, and similar disorders. One study published in the *Journal of Clinical Pharmacy and Therapeutics* showed the plant extract was effective at managing anxiety without the impact on job performance that exists with the traditional pharmaceuticals. Another study showed the herb was effective in reducing stress associated with undergoing surgery.

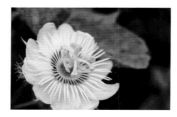

Herbal Power

MEDICINAL: Treats insomnia, fatigue, gastrointestinal issues, asthma, menopausal symptoms, irregular heartbeat, fibromyalgia, seizures, hemorrhoids, anxiety, stress, and nervousness; eases drug withdrawal.

COSMETIC: Improves health of the skin, hair, and scalp.

Application Methods

- Apply as an oil, salve, or tincture
- Drink as a tea

Precautions

Passionflower is generally considered safe with a few exceptions. Avoid if pregnant as the herb has been known to cause uterine contractions. Also avoid two to three weeks prior to surgery as it may increase the effects of anesthesia in the brain.

Other Names

Apricot Vine
Maypop
Purple Passion Flower
Water Lemon
Wild Passion Flower

Locating & Growing

Passionflower is pretty easy going when it comes to planting and doesn't really ask for much: some sunlight or partial shade, a warmish climate (though it's known to withstand Zone-5 winter temps), and moist soil.

RASPBERRY

RUBUS IDAEUS

Step aside chia, raspberry seeds and leaves are considered one of the hottest new superfoods around. It's no real surprise. They contain 83 percent essential fatty acids, vitamins E, B_1, and B_3, iron, calcium, magnesium, manganese, polyphenols, and UVA/UVB protection that rivals titanium oxide. Beauty enthusiasts are pretty psyched about raspberry's ability to erase acne scars, prevent and treat breakouts, reduce pores, smooth skin's surface, and even skin tone.

No raspberry leaves? Blackberry leaf makes an equally fantastic (and antioxidant-rich) substitution.

Did You Know?

Raspberry is widely known for its benefits in supporting pregnancy, labor, and delivery. Many cultures have used it to treat a wide range of ailments, including high blood pressure, kidney disorders, and infections. Topically, its leaves are a powerful disinfectant and are applied to wounds to speed healing.

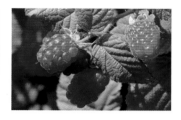

Herbal Power

MEDICINAL: Minimizes symptoms related to labor and delivery; eases morning sickness, muscle contractions, and uterine cramping; relieves sore throats; treats diarrhea; reduces fever.

COSMETIC: Fights acne, shrinks pores, smooths texture, evens skin tone; used as natural SPF in moisturizers, creams, and oils.

Application Methods

- Apply as a salve, oil, poultice, or compress
- Drink as a tea or tonic
- Use as a body splash, or in skincare

Precautions

Raspberry is considered safe and nontoxic.

Other Names

Framboise
Rubi Idaei Folium
Rubus

Locating & Growing

Raspberry bushes thrive in Zones 3 to 9 in areas with full sun, fertile, well-drained soil, and good air circulation. Don't plant near an area that grows or used to grow tomatoes, potatoes, peppers, eggplants, bramble berries, or roses, which can leave behind harmful diseases that can attack and destroy the fruit.

ROSEHIPS

ROSA CANINA

While this beautiful red fruit is revered for its vitamin C content, it's like a multivitamin grown on a plant, thanks to vitamins A, D, and E, essential fatty acids, and antioxidant-rich flavonoids. Eat them straight up off the stem to help with bladder infections, headaches, and more, or craft a DIY skin cream for a firm, youthful radiance.

Did You Know?

Rosehips are used to flavor teas and jellies, which is a good thing for your immune system. They have 20 times more vitamin C than oranges. While fresh rosehips are a major source of vitamin C, dried rosehips? Not so much. The act of drying the plant zaps a good bit of its C content.

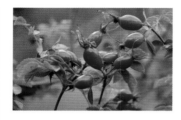

Herbal Power

MEDICINAL: Treats osteoarthritis, rheumatoid arthritis, menstrual cramps, fever, infections, stomach issues like diarrhea, cramps, and irritation; reduces cholesterol; prevents and treats colds; boosts immunity.

COSMETIC: Replenishes, repairs, and protects skin; evens skin tone; brightens; improves elasticity.

Application Methods

- Apply as a cream, oil, salve, face and body cleanser, or tincture
- Drink in a tea
- Use as a body wash, splash, or moisturizer

Precautions

While rosehips are considered safe, talk to your doctor before taking the herb as it may slow blood clotting, impact diabetes management, increase kidney stone risk, and impede the absorption of iron.

Other Names

Dog Rose
Hipberry
Persian Rose
Pink Rose

Locating & Growing

Rosehips, the seed pods of the rose plant, prefer light, sandy soil and loads of sunlight. To DIY like a pro, start with cuttings or seedlings and make some room for them to grow. Plants can top five feet when grown in conditions they love.

ROSEMARY

ROSMARINUS

Rosemary isn't just for seasoning lamb anymore. This widely studied herb features an active ingredient called carnosic acid, which has been shown in scientific studies to have serious protective effects in the brain. A recent study published in the *Journal of Neurochemistry* shows it protects brain cells from free radicals and may be used to treat neurodegenerative diseases like Parkinson's, Alzheimer's, and stroke. Researchers believe ongoing studies could show the herb to be a powerful treatment in anti-aging because of its ability to prevent disease, slow aging, and support the nervous system.

Did You Know?

Rosemary has a long and illustrious history as a multipurpose culinary and medicinal herb. Part of the mint family (along with basil, oregano, and lavender), it's been used for everything from gas relief and toothaches to baldness and memory loss. In the sixteenth century, doctors burnt rosemary in their sick rooms to disinfect the healing space and kill germs.

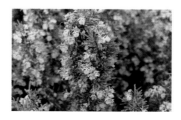

Herbal Power

MEDICINAL: Stimulates brain activity; enhances memory; eases headaches, migraines, depression, inflammation, and digestive issues, improves cardiovascular issues like low blood pressure and poor circulation; treats joint pain and inflammation; boosts mood; wards off illness.

COSMETIC: Conditions hair and skin in bath oils and hair tonics.

Application Methods

- Apply as a tincture, salve, ointment, poultice, compress, or essential oil
- Drink as a tea
- Use as a cleaning product

Precautions

It's safe to use with no toxicity reports during its long history of medicinal and culinary applications.

Other Names

Compass Plant
Old Man
Polar Plant
Romero

Locating & Growing

Rosemary is a somewhat high-maintenance plant. When it comes to water, not too much, not too little. When it comes to temperatures, not too hot, not too cold. In fact, it won't survive a freeze. It's often safest to keep the herb indoors in a brilliantly sunny spot with stable temperatures and soil dampness control.

SAGE

SALVIA OFFICINALIS

While there are many types of sage, *Salvia officinalis* is the most useful variety for your herbal medicine kit. Although there are many different types of sage within the same family, they have different benefits and uses. This particular sage—a.k.a. "common sage"—is widely used in aromatherapy as well as for wounds, infections, and cleaning solutions due to its antibacterial compounds.

Did You Know?

Sage has been present as a culinary herb for two thousand years. In ancient Greek and Roman times, royalty downed countless cups of sage tea believing it was a fountain of youth of sorts. During that same time, the herb was used both as a meat preservative and a memory booster. Later it was used for everything from snake bites to PMS to intestinal worms. In fact, sage was used during the Middle Ages to fight against the Black Death. Seems that these ancient civilizations were onto something. Research has since shown the herb to improve memory and fight against symptoms of Alzheimer's disease.

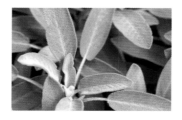

Herbal Power

MEDICINAL: Treats menstrual cramps, asthma, diarrhea, bloating, heartburn, depression, memory loss, gas, over-sweating, cold sores, gum disease, memory loss, menopause symptoms, and Alzheimer's disease.

COSMETIC: Refreshes scalp, masks gray hair, strengthens and shines hair; deodorizes teeth and body.

Application Methods

- Apply as a poultice, ointment, tonic, or tincture
- Drink as a tea or tonic
- Eat in food
- Use as a spray

Precautions

Sage contains the same active ingredient as in absinthe—thujone—so too much can be toxic. Experts suggest taking no more than 15 grams of leaves per dose. Nursing mothers should also avoid the herb as it can lower the benefits of breast milk.

Other Names

Garden Sage
Meadow Sage
Scarlet Sage
Spanish Sage
True Sage

Locating & Growing

This beautiful herb thrives in full sun and well-drained soils (no wet dirt for this guy). It grows best in Zones 4 to 8, blooms in June, and can handle drought conditions and rocky soil.

SELF-HEAL

A favorite in skincare lines because of its high vitamin C, vitamin K, thiamine, and tannin content, self-heal is known for its astringent, antiseptic, and anti-inflammatory benefits. It has roots in gourmet circles as well: Self-heal's leaves and stems (fresh or dried) can be the secret ingredient in your next farm-to-table salad or gourmet soup. Its fabulous purple flowers brighten up any bowl of greens without your guests having to know their first course is ultra-healing.

Did You Know?

The name "self-heal" comes from the fact that at one time this super herb was considered a panacea. It's used to treat Crohn's disease and other digestive issues, sexually transmitted diseases (STDs), and headaches, and the herb's high antioxidant content lends it potential in cancer and heart disease prevention as well as improved immunity. From a psychological perspective, it's taken to boost mood, raise energy levels, balance hormones, and awaken self-confidence and life force.

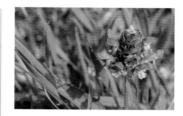

Herbal Power

MEDICINAL: Treats Crohn's disease, diarrhea, colic, gastroenteritis, throat issues, sore throat, fever, headache, liver disease, muscle spasms, STDs, and vaginal conditions.

COSMETIC: Fights inflammation and irritation; tightens pores.

Application Methods

- Apply as a splash, salve, ointment, or oil
- Use in a soap, mouthwash, or eye wash

Precautions

While no toxicity has been reported, herbalists suggest avoiding self-heal if you're pregnant or breastfeeding.

Other Names

All-Heal
Blue Curls
Brownwort
Carpenter's Herb
Heal-All
Hock-Heal
Sicklewort
Woundwort
Xia Ku Cao

Locating & Growing

Like many herbs with weed-like sensibilities, self-heal can grow just about anywhere, but it thrives in woods, meadows, and forest environments. Partial sun and mild temperatures are its sweet spot. If you're in a space with wet conditions, this herb spreads like wildfire.

SLIPPERY ELM

ULMUS RUBRA

Slippery elms, along with other elm trees, were wiped out by Dutch elm disease and are now considered endangered. This is partly due to their low numbers, but also to their slow-growing nature, which makes their population slow to replenish. You can find small and full-grown trees available in some nurseries as well as online, as their bark is still in demand. Many herbalists substitute marshmallow in recipes whenever allowed or readily available. A healthy tree can top 60 feet tall. What's coveted for medicinal use is the inner bark on the branches.

Did You Know?

Slippery elm is famous for its "mucilaginous" consistency, meaning the thick, gooey texture inherent in some plants. This viscosity, combined with its natural anti-inflammatory, anti-irritant characteristics, make it a soothing, nourishing ingredient in modern skincare lines. Back in the day, Native Americans used to soak slippery elm bark, cover wounds, and allow it to dry over the injured area as the bark imparted its healing compounds into the skin.

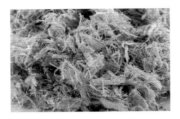

Herbal Power

MEDICINAL: Treats cough, sore throats, and laryngitis; eases digestive and GI (gastrointestinal) problems like constipation, diarrhea, IBS (irritable bowel syndrome), ulcers, and hemorrhoids; heals skin conditions like burns, cold sores, boils, ulcers, abscesses, and wounds; eases tooth pain.

COSMETIC: Soothes aging skin, combats wrinkles, erases sun damage.

Application Methods

- Apply as a compress or poultice
- Drink as a tea or infusion

Precautions

Don't take slippery elm if you're breastfeeding or pregnant. It's rumored to cause miscarriages and even trigger abortions. In some instances, slippery elm can cause an allergic reaction. If skin gets irritated, discontinue use or lower the dose.

Other Names

Indian Elm
Moose Elm
Orme
Red Elm
Sweet Elm

Locating & Growing

You'll find slippery elm in places with poorly drained soil like river beds, stream banks, low lands, mountain bottoms, or canyons. It's best suited for environments that allow for the tree to have moist soil and partial sunlight.

ST. JOHN'S WORT

HYPERICUM PERFORATUM

If you've taken any sort of road trip across the United States and Canada you've probably seen this herb growing abundantly on the side of the road. This herb is widely studied due to its powerful antifungal, antiviral, anticancer, and antibacterial properties. Research has shown it's able to suppress the AIDS virus, herpes virus, cancer proliferation, and more. Its striking buds are probably best known for their impact on feel-good neurotransmitters, including serotonin, noradrenaline, and dopamine, making it a powerful antidepressant remedy. (It takes three weeks of consistent use for its mood-boosting effects to kick in.)

Did You Know?

Hippocrates was a big fan of St. John's wort and recorded its uses in his medical records. It's natively European, but has proliferated pretty much everywhere. Australia, which now grows it as an exportable crop, produces 20 percent of the global supply.

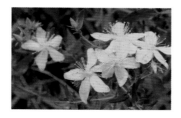

Herbal Power

MEDICINAL: Treats depression, stress, anxiety, shingles, herpes, sprains, wounds, burns, stings, and other injuries; eases symptoms of PMS and menopause; combats fatigue, loss of appetite, insomnia, muscle pain, seasonal affective disorder (SAD), obsessive-compulsive disorder (OCD), attention-deficit hyperactivity disorder (ADHD), mood swings, migraines, nerve pain, and irritable bowel syndrome (IBS); treats cancer, HIV/AIDS, and hepatitis C.

COSMETIC: Reduces stretch marks and helps eliminate bruises.

Application Methods

- Apply as a salve, ointment, poultice, tincture, or oil
- Drink as a tea

Precautions

St. John's wort should be used under the guidance of a doctor if you're pregnant or already taking antidepressants. Some people become sensitive to light when taking this herb. If this happens (skin becomes itchy, bumpy, red, inflamed), simply discontinue use or cut back on the dosage.

Other Names

Amber
Demon Chaser
Goatweed
Hardhay
Hypereikon
Klamath Weed
Millepertuis
Tipton Weed

Locating & Growing

Drench it, neglect it, shade it, or overexpose it to sun—St. John's wort doesn't care. It grows like a weed. Although it loves a sunny meadow in Zones 3 to 9, it sprouts easily and self-sows just about anywhere.

THYME

THYMUS VULGARIS

Packed with natural healing compounds—thymol, cineole, borneol, flavonoids, and tannins—this sweet-smelling, flowering beauty packs a powerful punch. Stash this herb in your medicine kit to fight everything from colds and flu symptoms to hair loss and funky breath. While you wouldn't expect to find this herb in your skincare regimen, its antiseptic, antibacterial, and astringent qualities make it a shoe-in for healing tough acne, preventing blemishes, tightening and toning skin, and deodorizing head to toe. Not bad for something you normally reserve for *herbes de Provence*.

Did You Know?

If thyme could talk, it'd tell you about how it was used by the Egyptians to mummify the dead, or how the Greeks gave it to their warriors to bolster courage. Because it's antiseptic, thyme was once used by doctors to clean wounds.

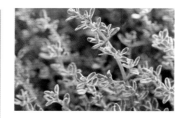

Herbal Power

MEDICINAL: Treats throat issues like bronchitis, sore throat, and whooping cough; soothes upset stomach, stomach cramps, gas, and diarrhea; kills parasites; kills germs that cause bad breath; stimulates appetite; stops tooth decay.

COSMETIC: Stimulates hair growth in blends made with rosemary and cedarwood; treats acne and foot odor.

Application Methods

- Apply as a salve, ointment, poultice, tincture, scrub, or oil
- Drink as a tea
- Eat in food
- Use as a cleaning product

Precautions

None. This herb is completely safe and nontoxic.

Other Names

Common Thyme
French Thyme
Garden Thyme
Red Thyme Oil
Rubbed Thyme
Spanish Thyme

Locating & Growing

Plant these seeds in spring (or anytime on your sill) in a sunny spot that's got moist, alkaline soil. Trim it often and it will love you.

VALERIAN

Valerian is teeming with good stuff: calcium; magnesium; vitamin B; caffeic, isovalerenic, and valerenic acids; essential oils; sesquiterpernes; and glycosides. It's most often considered "brain food" because its sweet spot is helping treat and support the nervous system.

Did You Know?

The earliest European colonists shipped valerian along with all of their belongings to start a new life in America. Because this herb is a natural stress and pain reliever that's easy to grow, packing it as a cure-all was a no-brainer.

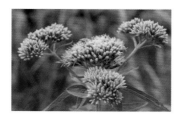

Herbal Power

MEDICINAL: Treats insomnia, stress, anxiety, headaches, nerve pain, depression, and nervous system issues; suppresses central nervous system activity; relaxes colon, uterus, and bronchial passages; relieves muscle and back tension; manages high blood pressure and irregular heartbeats.

COSMETIC: n/a

Application Methods

- Apply as a tincture, oil, poultice, or salve
- Drink as a tea

Precautions

Valerian is safe for short-term use (no studies have been done on the herb longer than one month). Side effects in some people can include insomnia, headache, anxiety, and a morning-after sluggishness or "hangover." You can't really overdose on it, but if your muscles or limbs start to feel heavy or sluggish, you may want to cut back the dosage.

Other Names

Common Valerian
Garden Heliotrope
Indian Valerian
Mexican Valerian
Pacific Valerian
Tagar

Locating & Growing

This perennial loves moist, rich soil and partial shade. Another self-sower, valerian will likely sprout up in abundance everywhere in your garden.

WITCH HAZEL

HAMAMELIS VIRGINIANA

Outdoor enthusiasts love the anti-itch, anti-inflammatory power of this wild shrub. Excellent for treating sunburn, bug bites, and bruises, you'll find it a necessary addition to backpacks and camping gear. Witch hazel is just as popular in beauty circles. Its eye brightening and astringent properties make it an excellent component in anti-aging skincare formulas and nourishing spa treatments. For everyday use, add it to a cotton ball and swipe over your face to fight acne, reduce fine lines and wrinkles, shrink pores, and remove makeup.

Did You Know?

Many people think these shrubs are actually trees because they grow up to 30 feet high and 15 feet wide. At one point, the shrub was called a "water witch" because its branches were used to locate underground water and mineral sources. Because they flower in the winter, they're often planted by people who need a visual mental boost or aromatherapeutic pick-me-up during the long winter months.

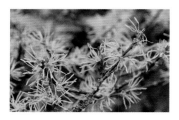

Herbal Power

MEDICINAL: Relieves itching, swelling, irritation, and pain related to skin conditions as well as hemorrhoids; treats diarrhea, colds, fever, varicose veins, and bruises; treats damaged gums, swimmer's ear, and sore throats; soothes diaper rash, stings, and bites; eases cramping and discomfort from menstruation.

COSMETIC: Heals eczema, soothes skin post-shave, and treats undereye bags and dark circles; works as an astringent, and treats varicose veins.

Application Methods

- Apply as a salve, ointment, or poultice
- Use as a splash or tonic

Precautions

Avoid using if skin is sunburnt, dry, overly sensitive, or windburned.

Other Names

Hazel
Snapping Tobacco Wood
Spotted Elder
Winter Bloom

Locating & Growing

Witch hazel shrubs are massive in both size and flower output. With gorgeous yellow flowers, ripe fruits, and burgeoning buds—often blooming at the same time—it's found quite often in forests or woodsy areas. Adaptable to sunlight and soil types, it's loved by herbalists and gardeners because of its color and sweet aroma.

Yarrow is one of the most fascinating herbs you'll find. Said to be a cure-all, it's been widely used around the world for centuries in a variety of modalities and cultures. It's best known for its dual nature. For example, it both triggers bleeding and stops bleeding. It makes sense because yarrow, like spearmint, is known to be "amphoteric," meaning that it moves to the location in or on your body where it's needed. At the same time, it's stimulating and calming depending on the patient's needs. Even more fascinating, it works almost immediately, particularly when reducing swelling or stopping bleeding, and takes down high fevers in record time (that's because it's also diaphoretic and triggers sweating).

Did You Know?

Yarrow is named after Achilles, the Greek Trojan War leader, who used it during battle. He bound his warriors' feet in the herb to stop bleeding and heal their wounds more quickly.

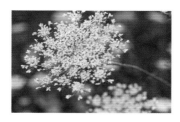

Herbal Power

MEDICINAL: Heals bruises, wounds, and sprains; reduces inflammation; slows and stops bleeding; regulates menstrual cycles, triggers late periods, eases cramps and other PMS (premenstrual syndrome) symptoms; reduces fever; lessens bloating, gas, stomach cramps, and related GI issues; triggers hunger and appetite; supports liver functions.

COSMETIC: n/a

Application Methods

- Apply as a salve or poultice
- Drink as a tea
- Use as an oil or tincture

Precautions

Yarrow is considered safe and nontoxic; however, because of its effects on bleeding, cramping, and uterine muscles, pregnant women should avoid using it.

Other names

Bloodwort
Carpenter's Weed
Devil's Nettle
Erba Da Falegname
Gandana
Schafgarbe
Milefolio
Staunchweed
Wound Wort

Locating & Growing

This is one-stop seeding. Plant yarrow in your garden once; it will grow easily, thrive in moist soil and full sunlight, and, best of all, will self-sow. Like its effects in your body, yarrow is highly adaptable to nearly any growing conditions.

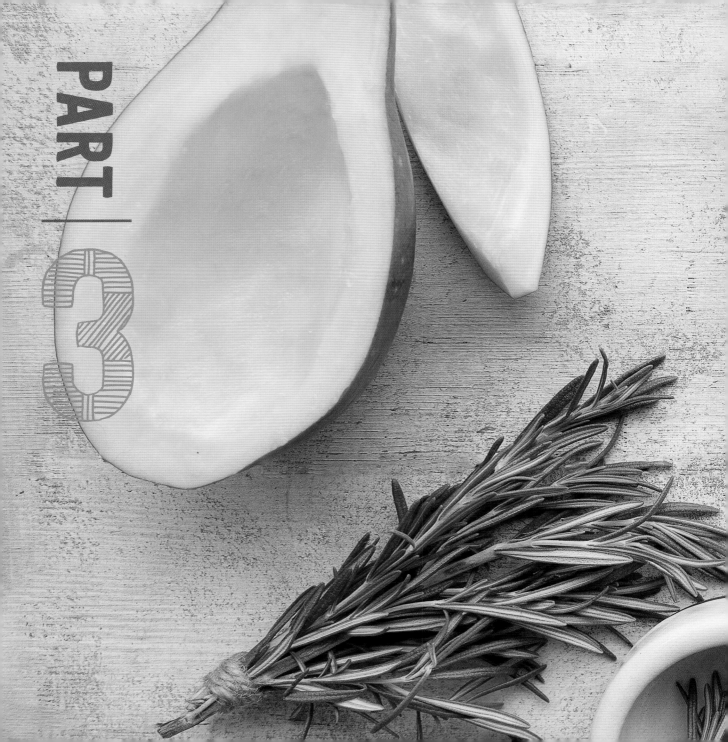

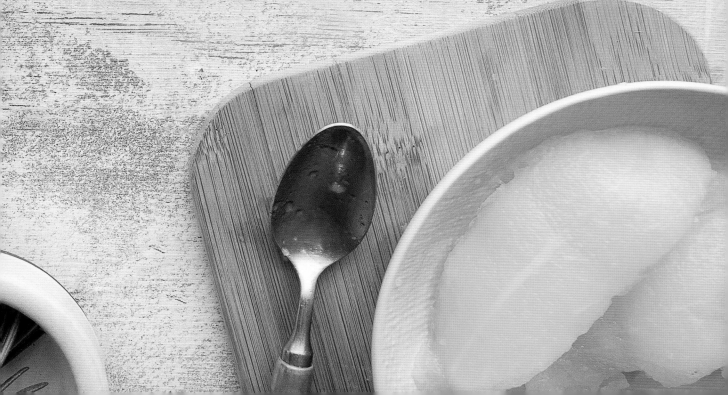

PART 3

THE REMEDIES

(Plus a Few Products)

Treatments in these chapters address everything from oily hair and body odor to serious ailments like UTIs and migraines. Remedies are also included for anxiety, depression, insomnia, and other conditions so important to overall wellness. Finally, this section wraps with a handful of go-to remedies for natural home cleaning products and self-treatments for the day after some of the most common non-medical issues we encounter.

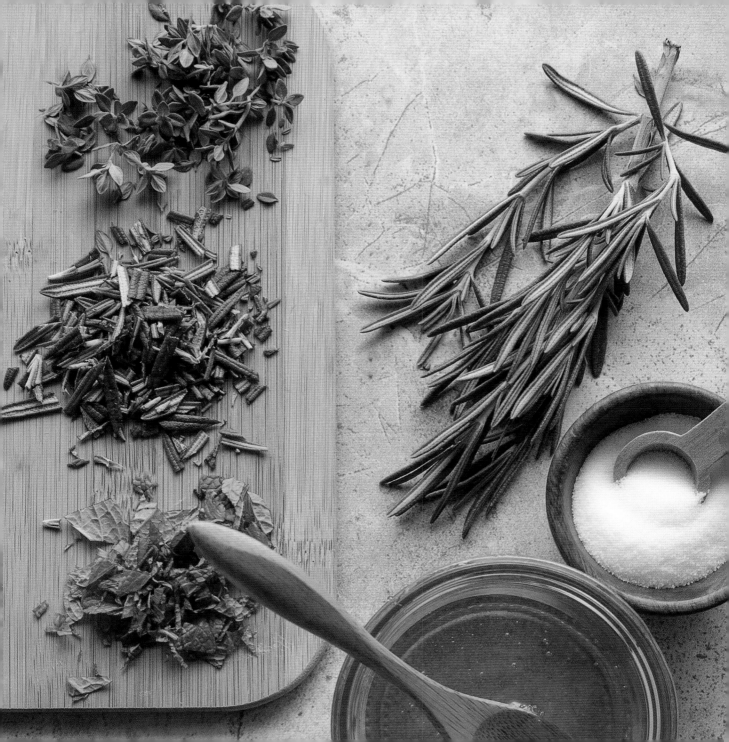

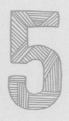

FACE AND HAIR CARE

ACNE

Your teen years are behind you, so what's with the persisting acne? Unfortunately, acne will rear its ugly head (and whitehead and blackhead) whenever oil and dead skin cells clog fragile pores. You may already know that scrubbing too hard, using harsh chemicals, and picking at them can make the issue worse. Mild and gentle, the herbs used to treat acne can address inflammation, help clear up pimples, and minimize scarring. Use alone or alongside other treatments.

Soothing Aloe Vera and Calendula Facial

YIELD: 1 TREATMENT
STORAGE: NOT RECOMMENDED
TIME: 10 MINUTES

Calendula is a gentle astringent that eliminates bacteria while easing inflammation. This soothing facial stops redness and relieves discomfort while restoring skin's balance and improving your complexion.

½ teaspoon alcohol-free aloe vera gel
½ teaspoon calendula oil
1 drop chamomile essential oil

1. In a small dish, combine the aloe vera gel, calendula oil, and chamomile essential oil.
2. Using your fingertips, apply a thin layer to your freshly washed face.
3. Leave in place for 5 to 10 minutes.
4. Rinse your face with cool water and pat dry. Follow up with your favorite oil-free moisturizer if needed.
5. Repeat this treatment once daily while acne persists.

Juniper Berry-Lavender Toner

YIELD: 30 TREATMENTS
STORAGE: DARK-COLORED GLASS BOTTLE
TIME: 5 MINUTES

This facial toner is simple but powerful. The essential oils offer a pleasant aroma, plus they are powerful antiseptics that stimulate your circulation and help damaged skin heal.

½ cup alcohol-free witch hazel extract
4 drops juniper berry essential oil
4 drops lavender essential oil

1. In a dark-colored glass bottle, combine the witch hazel extract, juniper berry essential oil, and lavender essential oil.
2. Cap tightly and shake well.
3. Using a cotton ball, apply a thin layer to your freshly washed face. Follow up with oil-free moisturizer.
4. Use this toner morning and evening. Store in a cool, dark place.

Rosemary-Mint Facial Scrub

YIELD: 1 TREATMENT
STORAGE: NOT RECOMMENDED
TIME: 10 MINUTES

By exfoliating gently, this facial scrub helps to unblock clogged pores. The white wine and honey soften skin and the rosemary stimulates cell renewal. Use this scrub to stop acne outbreaks fast.

½ teaspoon chopped mint leaves
½ teaspoon rosemary leaves
½ teaspoon thyme leaves
2 tablespoons white wine
1 teaspoon honey
2 teaspoons fine sea salt

1. In a small saucepan, combine the mint, rosemary, thyme, white wine, and honey.
2. Turn the heat to medium-high and bring to a simmer.
3. Reduce the heat to medium-low and simmer for 10 minutes or until the volume has been reduced by half.
4. Allow the mixture to cool completely.
5. Transfer the liquid to a small glass bowl.
6. Add the sea salt and stir gently.
7. Using gentle circular motions, apply the scrub to your freshly washed face.
8. Leave in place for 5 to 10 minutes.
9. Rinse your face with cool water and pat dry. Follow up with oil-free moisturizer.
10. Use this scrub twice weekly during acne breakouts.

CHAPPED LIPS

Regardless of whether you spend lots of time inside or outside, chapped lips plague just about everyone at some point. Blame sunburn, or wind, or dry indoor air. While there is no shortage of commercial remedies available, home remedies made with herbs can help protect delicate lip tissue and heal chapped lips quickly. Do your best to stay out of extreme cold and direct sunlight until your lips are smooth again.

Chamomile Lip Scrub

YIELD: 10 TREATMENTS
STORAGE: SMALL GLASS JAR
TIME: 5 MINUTES

This four-ingredient lip scrub gently exfoliates, revealing new skin and allowing moisture to penetrate where it's needed most. Nourishing chamomile essential oil helps ease the discomfort associated with inflammation, dryness, and cracked skin.

1 teaspoon alcohol-free aloe vera gel
1 teaspoon honey
2 drops chamomile essential oil
1 teaspoon sugar

1. In a small jar, combine the aloe vera gel, honey, and chamomile essential oil.
2. Add the sugar and stir thoroughly.
3. With a fingertip, apply a dab of the scrub to your lips.
4. Using gentle circular motions, lightly scrub for 10 seconds.
5. Rinse your lips with cool water. Follow up with moisturizing lip balm.
6. Repeat this treatment 1 or 2 times daily while suffering from chapped lips. Store in a cool, dark place.

Lavender-Geranium
Lip Balm

YIELD: 30 TREATMENTS
STORAGE: SMALL GLASS JAR
TIME: 10 MINUTES

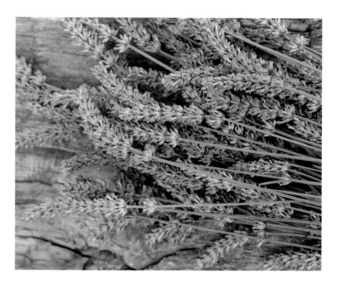

You'll love how silky soft your lips feel as this healing balm boosts hydration and soothes irritation. The lavender and geranium essential oils help damaged skin heal while leaving a hint of pleasant fragrance.

1 tablespoon beeswax
1 tablespoon coconut oil
1 teaspoon calendula oil
2 drops lavender essential oil
1 drop geranium essential oil

1. In a double boiler, combine the beeswax and coconut oil over low heat.
2. Stir gently until the beeswax has melted completely.
3. Remove from the heat and add the calendula oil. Stir well.
4. Add the lavender and geranium essential oils and stir well.
5. Pour the balm into a small jar and cool completely.
6. Using your index finger, apply a thin layer to your lips.
7. Use this balm as often as you like. Store in a cool, dark place.

♥ While this balm helps heal chapped lips, it also works well for dry knees and elbows.

COLOR-DAMAGED HAIR

Whether you've lightened your hair or gone a few shades darker, it's likely that all those dyes that gave your locks luscious color also left them with some dryness, breakage, or frizz. While the only way to permanently eliminate chemical damage like the kind that comes from relaxers, perms, and hair color is to cut your hair, these nourishing herbal remedies can smooth cuticles, repair ends, and hydrate thirsty tresses so hair gets back on the road to health.

Aloe Vera–Peppermint Hair Mask

YIELD: 1 TREATMENT
STORAGE: NOT RECOMMENDED
TIME: 20 MINUTES

Aloe vera provides the moisture that dehydrated or damaged locks so desperately need, while jojoba oil adds shine, and peppermint essential oil stimulates circulation in your scalp (read: helps new hair grow).

1 tablespoon alcohol-free aloe vera gel
1 tablespoon jojoba oil
6 drops peppermint essential oil

1. In a small bowl, combine the aloe vera gel, jojoba oil, and peppermint essential oil.
2. Apply the entire treatment to your hair and scalp, massaging well.
3. Place a disposable shower cap on your head and leave the treatment in place for 15 minutes.
4. When finished, wash and condition your hair as usual.
5. Use once or twice weekly for best results.

Chamomile Conditioner

YIELD: 1 TREATMENT
STORAGE: NOT RECOMMENDED
TIME: 20 MINUTES

Conditioning chamomile and fortifying egg protein are the dynamic duo in this shine booster and strand strengthener. Bonus: It reduces tangles and prevents future breakage, too. Dampen hair before using this treatment.

1 egg yolk, beaten
1 teaspoon sunflower oil
4 drops chamomile essential oil

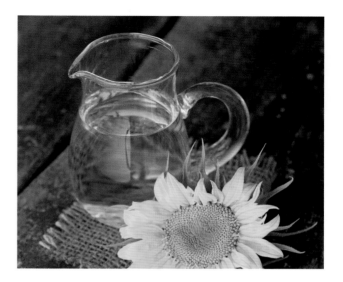

1. In a small bowl, combine the egg yolk, sunflower oil, and chamomile essential oil.
2. Beat vigorously to combine.
3. Massage the entire treatment into your hair and scalp.
4. Leave in place for 15 minutes.
5. When finished, rinse your hair thoroughly with cool water. Follow up with your favorite shampoo and conditioner.
6. Use at least once weekly for best results.

CROW'S FEET & LAUGH LINES

Crow's feet and laugh lines don't have to be an inevitable sign of aging skin. While these little wrinkles are the natural result of our daily facial expressions (including, but not limited to, smiling and laughing), you can soften them and prevent them from becoming deeper by wearing sunscreen daily, applying weekly hydrating masks, and nourishing your skin with nutrient-dense moisturizers. Smile and give these remedies a try. Use them regularly and your skin will stay young-looking longer.

Rosemary-Papaya Facial Mask

YIELD: 1 TREATMENT
STORAGE: NOT RECOMMENDED
TIME: 20 MINUTES

Ready to get your glow back? Fresh papaya contains vitamin C to stimulate collagen production, as well as papain, an enzyme that exfoliates and tightens pores. Rosemary essential oil speeds cell renewal and improves circulation.

¼ cup puréed fresh papaya
6 drops rosemary essential oil

1. In a small bowl, combine the papaya and rosemary essential oil.
2. Using your fingertips, apply the mixture to your freshly washed face, focusing on crow's feet and laugh lines.
3. Relax for 15 minutes. If the mixture seems too slippery, keep it in place by covering your face with a paper or cotton facial mask.
4. When finished, rinse your face with cool water and apply your favorite moisturizer.
5. You may feel a tingling sensation while this mask is doing its work. If you experience discomfort, stop the treatment.

Frankincense-Lavender Skin Serum

YIELD: 2 OUNCES
STORAGE: DARK-COLORED GLASS BOTTLE WITH DROPPER
TIME: 5 MINUTES

This light herbal serum offers a powerhouse of age-defying oils. Macadamia rejuvenates tired, aging skin. Lavender calms and moisturizes. Meadowfoam delivers major antioxidants. And frankincense balances pH while repairing skin cells.

2 tablespoons macadamia nut oil
1½ tablespoons meadowfoam seed oil
15 drops frankincense essential oil
10 drops lavender essential oil

1. Add all the ingredients to a dark-colored glass bottle fitted with a glass dropper.
2. Shake for 30 seconds to blend.
3. With your fingertips, apply a thin layer to your skin, focusing on crow's feet and laugh lines.
4. Let the serum absorb into your skin. Follow up with your favorite moisturizer.
5. You can use this serum to hydrate your entire face if you like. Store it in a cool, dark place.

Lavender Toner with Vitamins C and E

YIELD: ABOUT 2 OUNCES
STORAGE: DARK-COLORED GLASS BOTTLE
TIME: 10 MINUTES

This fragrant toner nourishes skin and provides a lightweight layer of protective moisture. With daily use, it reduces the appearance of crow's feet, or dry, indoor-air-damaged skin.

1¾ ounces rose hydrosol
¾ teaspoon vitamin C crystals
20 drops lavender essential oil
20 drops vitamin E oil

1. In a small bowl, combine the rose hydrosol and vitamin C crystals.
2. Stir gently until the vitamin C crystals are dissolved.
3. Using a funnel, transfer the liquid to a dark-colored glass bottle.
4. Carefully add the lavender essential oil and vitamin E oil to the bottle.
5. Shake well.
6. Using a cotton ball, apply a few drops to your clean face. Follow up with your favorite moisturizer.
7. Use this toner each morning and night. Store in a cool, dark place.

DANDRUFF

Don't toss out that black sweater just yet. There are easy, effective ways to deal with annoying dandruff, which can be caused by everything from a dry, overly oily, or under-shampooed scalp to skin conditions like eczema, psoriasis, or fungus. Treatments like the ones here make it simple to control both the side effects and the underlying causes of the problem.

Ginger-Tea Tree Scalp Tonic

YIELD: 1 TREATMENT
STORAGE: NOT RECOMMENDED
TIME: 20 MINUTES

Ginger's anti-inflammatory action eases the itching associated with dandruff. Olive oil imparts natural moisture to dry, flaky skin. Tea tree essential oil lends a hand by killing fungus.

1 palm-sized piece of fresh ginger root, peeled
1 tablespoon olive oil
2 drops tea tree essential oil

1. Use a garlic press or juicer to extract as much juice from the ginger root as you can. If using a garlic press, grate the ginger before pressing it.
2. In a small bowl, mix the juice, olive oil, and tea tree essential oil together.
3. Wet your hair and apply the entire remedy to the scalp.
4. Massage gently.
5. Leave the treatment in place for 15 minutes.
6. When finished, rinse your hair thoroughly with cool water. Follow up with your favorite shampoo and conditioner.
7. Repeat this treatment 2 to 3 times weekly until the dandruff is gone. If you use a hair dryer, avoid exposing your scalp to high heat, as it slows the healing process.

Herbal Dandruff Shampoo

YIELD: 15 TREATMENTS
STORAGE: SHAMPOO BOTTLE
TIME: 30 MINUTES

This natural dandruff shampoo is a fantastic alternative to commercial preparations thanks to a cocktail of high-powered, antioxidant-rich herbs that heal the scalp sans the signature medicinal scent of over-the-counter options.

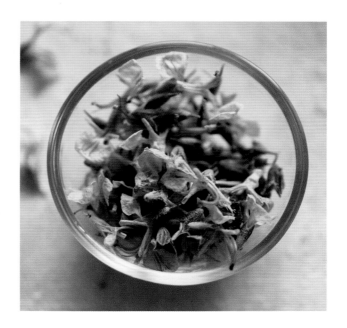

- **1 cup water**
- **1 heaping tablespoon dried lavender**
- **1 heaping tablespoon dried mint**
- **1 heaping tablespoon dried rosemary**
- **⅓ cup liquid castile soap**
- **¼ teaspoon almond or olive oil**
- **5 drops eucalyptus essential oil**
- **5 drops tea tree essential oil**

1. In a small saucepan, bring the water to a boil.
2. Add the lavender, mint, and rosemary, cover the pan, and reduce the heat to low. Simmer for 20 minutes.
3. Strain the mixture into a bowl and let it cool.
4. Add the castile soap and mix gently.
5. Add the almond oil and eucalyptus and tea tree essential oils.
6. Mix gently, then use a funnel to transfer the shampoo to a bottle.
7. Shampoo and follow up with your favorite conditioner.
8. Style as usual, avoiding high heat from the blow dryer.
9. Use daily whenever dandruff is a problem. Store in the shower.

DRY SKIN

The only upside to dry skin is that it comes with a somewhat simple solution. Because dryness is caused by a lack of hydration in the skin's upper layer, natural oils and herbs work brilliantly to rejuvenate, rehydrate, and moisturize cells. Try these fast and easy treatments on other problem areas like elbows and knees, too. (And if you're exposed to an arid climate or dry indoors, use a humidifier at night.)

Honey Moisture Mask with Hyssop and Lavender

YIELD: 1 TREATMENT
STORAGE: NOT RECOMMENDED
TIME: 15 MINUTES

This trio of skin saviors—hyssop, lavender, and honey—soothes irritation, nourishes parched cells, and calms inflammation. Over-the-counter aloe vera gel is a great substitution if you don't have an aloe vera plant.

1 aloe vera leaf or 1 teaspoon store-bought alcohol-free aloe vera gel
1 teaspoon honey, warmed
1 teaspoon finely chopped fresh hyssop leaves
2 drops lavender essential oil

1. Split the aloe vera leaf open lengthwise and scoop out the aloe vera gel.
2. In a small bowl, combine the aloe vera gel with the honey.
3. Using a fork or a small whisk, stir well.
4. Add the hyssop leaves and lavender essential oil.
5. Stir again to blend all the ingredients.
6. Using your fingertips, apply the entire mask to your face and neck.
7. Lie back and relax for at least 10 to 15 minutes.
8. Rinse your face with cool water when finished. Follow up with your favorite moisturizer.
9. Enjoy twice weekly for best results.

Rich Chamomile Facial Cream

YIELD: 30 TREATMENTS
STORAGE: GLASS JAR
TIME: 20 MINUTES

With rich oils and beeswax for a smooth, supple feel, this moisturizer makes the most of chamomile's healing ability.

1 teaspoon dried chamomile flowers
½ cup boiling water
3 tablespoons almond oil
3 tablespoons avocado oil
1 tablespoon jojoba oil
1 ounce beeswax
2 teaspoons glycerin
10 drops chamomile essential oil
10 drops geranium essential oil

1. In a small bowl, combine the chamomile flowers and boiling water. Cover the bowl and steep for 15 minutes.
2. Meanwhile, in the top of a double boiler, combine the almond, avocado, and jojoba oils.
3. Add the beeswax to the oils and stir over low heat until melted.
4. Strain the chamomile-infused water, being careful to keep flower bits out of the liquid. Measure 1 ounce of the infusion. Discard any unused portion. ▶
5. Transfer the oil mixture to a medium glass bowl. One drop at a time, add the chamomile infusion to the oil mixture, stirring with a small whisk until it thickens and cools.
6. Add the glycerin and mix thoroughly. Add the chamomile and geranium essential oils and mix again.
7. Transfer the cream to a glass jar with a tight-fitting lid.
8. With your fingertips, massage a small amount onto your freshly washed face, neck, and chest.
9. Use nightly before bed. Store in a cool, dark place.

DULL, DRY HAIR

Dull, dry tresses occur when brittle hair shafts are unable to absorb or retain the moisture that's necessary for a lush, radiant mane. It's true, harsh chemicals and heated styling tools are part of the problem, but you can minimize their impact and restore strand health with remedies that lock out heat, seal in hydration, and restore vitality.

Rosemary Hair Balm

YIELD: 1 TREATMENT
STORAGE: NOT RECOMMENDED
TIME: 15 MINUTES

The protein in gelatin fortifies damaged hair, while apple cider vinegar and rosemary give it lustrous shine. Prepare this treatment just before you shampoo.

1 cup hot tap water
1 tablespoon unflavored gelatin
1 teaspoon apple cider vinegar
5 drops rosemary essential oil

1. In a small bowl, combine the tap water and gelatin, whisking to blend well.
2. Set the mixture aside for about 5 minutes.
3. Once it begins to gel slightly, add the apple cider vinegar and rosemary essential oil.
4. Stir well to combine.
5. Work through your freshly shampooed hair and onto your scalp.
6. Leave the balm in place for 10 minutes.
7. Rinse with warm water.
8. Repeat once or twice weekly for best results.

Lavender Hair Mask

YIELD: 1 TREATMENT
STORAGE: NOT RECOMMENDED
TIME: 20 MINUTES

Yogurt, honey, and rich oils infuse protein and moisture into parched hair, repairing damage while amping up shine. Prepare this treatment just before you shampoo.

¼ cup plain yogurt
1 tablespoon honey
1 tablespoon olive or sunflower oil
5 drops lavender essential oil

1. In a blender, combine all the ingredients.
2. Process on medium-low speed until blended.
3. Transfer to a plastic squeeze bottle.
4. Work the treatment through your freshly shampooed hair and massage into your scalp.
5. Leave the mask in place for 15 minutes.
6. Rinse with warm water.
7. Use twice weekly for best results.

Floral Hot Oil Infusion

YIELD: 1 TREATMENT
STORAGE: NOT RECOMMENDED
TIME: 45 MINUTES

There's a reason hot oil treatments are time-honored salon favorites. They strengthen brittle hair, add shine, and restore moisture. No sunflower oil, no problem. Olive or corn oil works wonders.

¼ cup sunflower oil
1 tablespoon lavender flowers
1 tablespoon chopped rosemary leaves

1. In a small saucepan, add the sunflower oil, lavender, and rosemary. Heat over low heat for 30 minutes.
2. Strain the oil into a bowl, then use a funnel to transfer it to a plastic squeeze bottle.
3. When comfortably warm to touch, apply the entire treatment to your hair and scalp, gently massaging it in.
4. Wrap your head in a damp, hot towel.
5. Leave the infusion in place for 15 minutes.
6. Shampoo and condition as usual.
7. Use once or twice weekly for best results.

ECZEMA OF THE FACE

Thanks to inflammation, reddening, and irritation, facial eczema is not just uncomfortable, it's also hard to hide. Because so many underlying factors can trigger this condition, your first step is to work with your doctor to determine why it's happening so you can treat the root cause effectively. In the meantime, use herbal remedies to soothe your symptoms.

Soothing Calendula-Carrot Facial Mask

YIELD: 1 TREATMENT
STORAGE: NOT RECOMMENDED
TIME: 30 MINUTES

Calendula oil and carrot seed essential oil come together to soothe and moisturize irritated skin. The carrots and honey in this recipe are natural antiseptics that leave skin feeling fresh and healthy.

1 organic carrot, boiled and mashed
1 teaspoon raw honey
5 drops calendula oil
3 drops carrot seed essential oil

1. In a small bowl, combine the carrot and raw honey, mixing until smooth.
2. Add the calendula oil and carrot seed essential oil, mixing again to incorporate.
3. Using your fingertips, apply the mask to your freshly washed face.
4. Relax for 15 to 20 minutes.
5. Rinse your face with cool water when finished. Follow up with your favorite moisturizer.
6. Use 2 to 3 times weekly.

Chamomile Facial Compress

YIELD: 1 TREATMENT
STORAGE: NOT RECOMMENDED
TIME: 15 MINUTES

Instant relief! This soothing compress is a simple remedy that eases discomfort quickly. Chamomile essential oil helps stop inflammation and itching while promoting faster healing.

½ cup hot tap water
1 teaspoon coconut oil
6 drops chamomile essential oil

1. In a shallow bowl, combine the hot tap water and coconut oil.
2. Add the chamomile essential oil and stir.
3. Soak a soft cloth with the mixture and squeeze out the excess liquid.
4. Place the cloth over your face and rest for 15 minutes, refreshing the cloth with the warm solution each time it cools.
5. Apply once or twice daily. Use for as many days as eczema persists.

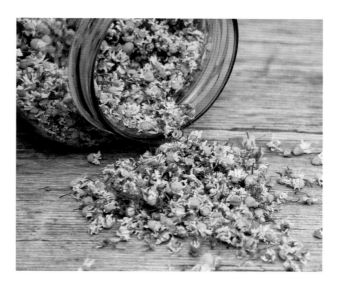

OILY HAIR

If your strands get that stringy, midday cling despite daily washing, you're not alone—but there's not much solace in being part of the oily crowd. Shampooing each day is just part of the solution. Keep oiliness at bay with easy-to-make toners and rinses that leave locks soft, shiny, and grease-free. Remember to condition just the ends of your hair to keep buildup from forming.

Rosemary-Lemon Rinse

YIELD: 1 TREATMENT
STORAGE: NOT RECOMMENDED
TIME: 5 MINUTES

Rosemary and lemon essential oils and apple cider vinegar cut through excess oil, nourish your scalp, and leave hair looking fresh. Other oils to try? Tea tree, peppermint, lavender, or sage work beautifully, too!

½ cup water
2 tablespoons apple cider vinegar
4 drops rosemary essential oil
2 drops lemon essential oil

1. In a plastic squeeze bottle, combine the water, apple cider vinegar, and rosemary and lemon essential oils.
2. Just before use, place your index finger over the bottle's tip and shake well.
3. After shampooing, apply the entire treatment to your scalp. Do not rinse.
4. Gently squeeze any excess solution from your hair. Apply a little conditioner to the ends if needed.
5. Towel your hair dry afterward and style it as usual.

Witch Hazel Scalp Toner

YIELD: 4 OUNCES
STORAGE: PLASTIC SQUEEZE BOTTLE
TIME: 5 MINUTES

Witch hazel is a stylist's secret weapon thanks to astringent compounds that cut through scalp oil effortlessly. Lavender essential oil leaves an intoxicating fragrance that helps you forget this is a treatment. Mix it up with other oils like tea tree, sage, lemon, or peppermint.

4 ounces alcohol-free witch hazel extract
1 teaspoon lavender essential oil

1. In a plastic squeeze bottle, combine the witch hazel extract and lavender essential oil.
2. Just before use, place your index finger over the bottle's tip and shake well.
3. After washing your hair, apply enough of the entire treatment to moisten your scalp. Do not rinse.
4. Gently squeeze any excess solution from your hair. Apply a little conditioner to the ends if needed.
5. Towel your hair dry afterward and style it as usual.
6. Use daily. Store in a cool, dark place.

♥ If you find that your scalp is becoming too dry, use the treatment every other day or try one made with apple cider vinegar instead of witch hazel extract.

Lavender-Rosemary Dry Shampoo

YIELD: ABOUT 1 CUP
STORAGE: SUGAR SHAKER
TIME: 10 MINUTES

This dry shampoo refreshes tresses when you don't have time to lather up. If you have dark hair, add the optional cinnamon or unsweetened cocoa powder to disguise any cornstarch that brushing fails to remove.

½ cup cornstarch
¼ cup baking soda
2 tablespoons ground cinnamon or unsweetened cocoa powder (optional for dark hair)
2 drops lavender essential oil
2 drops rosemary essential oil

1. In a large bowl, add the cornstarch, baking soda, and ground cinnamon (if using). Blend using a whisk or a fork.
2. Add the lavender and rosemary essential oils 1 drop at a time, whisking thoroughly after each addition.
3. Using a spoon and funnel, transfer the shampoo to a sugar shaker.
4. Section your hair and shake a small amount of the dry shampoo onto the roots.
5. Lightly massage with your fingertips.
6. Brush vigorously to remove.
7. Use when needed. Store in a cool, dry place.

♥ To add volume, flip your head upside down and massage again. Brush your hair while your head is upside down, and brush a second time with your head in its normal position.

PUFFY EYES

Sure, drinking binges, crying jags, late nights, and seasonal allergies can all cause pretty major bags under your eyes, but redness and puffiness don't need to be the first things other people see. Use these herbal remedies to bring down the swelling and improve your outlook on life.

Lavender-Lemon Bedtime Serum

YIELD: ABOUT 1 OUNCE
STORAGE: DARK-COLORED SMALL GLASS BOTTLE
TIME: 5 MINUTES

Let this magical de-puffer work while you sleep. Lavender and lemon essential oils help alleviate swollen under-eye tissue. Almond oil adds moisture, smoothing the appearance of delicate skin.

1 ounce almond oil
10 drops lavender essential oil
10 drops lemon essential oil

1. In a dark-colored glass bottle, add the almond oil and the lavender and lemon essential oils and shake well.
2. Using your fingertips, gently dab 1 or 2 drops of serum to the area under each eye.
3. Use nightly before bed. Store in a cool, dark place.

♟ Elevate your head with an extra pillow. Sleep on your back to help prevent fluid from accumulating in the tissue beneath your eyes.

Cool Chamomile Toner

YIELD: ABOUT 2 OUNCES
STORAGE: DARK-COLORED SMALL GLASS BOTTLE
TIME: 5 MINUTES

This chamomile–witch hazel combo creates an amazing astringent that tightens tissue, reduces swelling, and eases inflammation. It isn't necessary to refrigerate this toner, but using it cold shrinks swelling more than applying the toner at room temperature.

2 ounces alcohol-free witch hazel extract
4 drops chamomile essential oil

1. In a dark-colored glass bottle, combine the witch hazel extract with the chamomile essential oil.
2. Shake well before each use.
3. Using a cotton ball, apply 2 to 3 drops of toner to the area under each eye.

♥ If you have a little time, lie back and rest for 5 to 10 minutes after application, placing a cloth under your eyes and topping the cloth with an ice cube beneath each eye.

Rosemary Under-Eye Balm

YIELD: ABOUT 1 OUNCE
STORAGE: DARK-COLORED SMALL GLASS BOTTLE
TIME: 5 MINUTES

Rosemary essential oil acts as a mild diuretic, which reduces under-eye swelling. It also contains anti-inflammatory compounds that help lighten discoloration and nutrients that bolster compromised capillaries.

2 tablespoons argan oil
7 drops rosemary essential oil

1. In a dark-colored glass bottle, combine the argan oil and rosemary essential oil.
2. Shake well to combine.
3. Using your fingertips, apply 1 to 2 drops to the under-eye area.
4. This treatment is suitable for daily use and can be applied morning and night. Store in a cool, dark place.

♥ Allow a few minutes for absorption before using other treatments or cosmetics.

ROSACEA

The redness, swelling, and inflamed, irritated patches associated with rosacea often leave sufferers desperate for a treatment that brings this incurable condition under control. Instead of paying top dollar for expensive chemical-based solutions, try this roundup of herbs, proven to erase and/or minimize hard-to-banish symptoms. With minimal side effects, surprising efficacy, and tiny price tags, these remedies ease irritation while moisturizing your skin and alleviating discoloration.

Gentle Chamomile Facial Toner

YIELD: ABOUT ½ CUP
STORAGE: GLASS JAR
TIME: 30 MINUTES

With terpene bisabolol, a natural pain and inflammation reliever, chamomile balances troubled skin, easing discomfort and redness. Make a new batch of this toner every few days so you always have some on hand.

1 cup water
1 handful dried chamomile flowers or
** 3 handfuls fresh chamomile flowers**

1. In a small saucepan, combine the water and chamomile. On high heat, bring to a boil.
2. Reduce the heat to low and simmer the chamomile for 15 minutes or until the volume of the water has been reduced by about half.
3. Cool completely and strain the chamomile infusion into a glass jar.
4. To apply the solution, soak a cotton ball and spread a thin layer over your freshly washed face.
5. Let the toner dry naturally before applying your favorite moisturizer.
6. Use once or twice daily. Store in the refrigerator.

Lavender-Aloe Vera Moisturizer

YIELD: ABOUT 1 OUNCE
STORAGE: SMALL GLASS JAR
TIME: 5 MINUTES

Lavender and aloe vera make an extremely effective healing duo with their natural antiseptic, anti-inflammatory, and soothing power. Keep this oil-free moisturizer refrigerated if you use fresh aloe vera gel rather than the pre-packaged kind.

2 tablespoons alcohol-free aloe vera gel
8 drops lavender essential oil

1. In a small bowl, add the aloe vera gel and lavender essential oil. Using a whisk or fork, mix until thoroughly blended.
2. Transfer the moisturizer to a glass jar with a tight-fitting lid.
3. Using your fingertips, apply a thin layer of moisturizer to your face, neck, and chest.
4. Let it absorb completely before applying any other products.
5. Use once or twice daily.

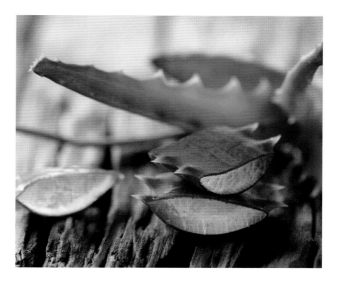

SPLIT ENDS

While the only way to get rid of split ends for good is to have them trimmed off, there are some easy ways to smooth them down so your hair looks less frazzled. Speed the healing time of dry, damaged locks by avoiding hot styling tools, salt water, and chemicals such as those found in home hair-color kits. They make the problem worse—and your herbal remedies have to work twice as hard!

Geranium-Honey Hair Repair

YIELD: 1 TREATMENT
STORAGE: NOT RECOMMENDED
TIME: 20 MINUTES

With honey and olive oil to moisturize, this nourishing treatment also contains geranium essential oil to strengthen hair. Use between haircuts to fortify strands and preserve that healthy, freshly cut salon look.

1 tablespoon olive oil
1 tablespoon honey
3 drops geranium essential oil

1. In a small glass bowl, combine the olive oil and honey.
2. Microwave on low power for 15 seconds.
3. Stir the honey and olive oil together. If not quite warm enough, repeat step 2.
4. Add the geranium essential oil.
5. Dampen your hair and apply the entire treatment.
6. Cover your head with a disposable shower cap, then wrap it with a towel.
7. Leave the hair repair in place for 10 to 15 minutes, then wash, condition, and style as usual.
8. Repeat once or twice weekly.

Rosemary-Aloe Vera Leave-In Conditioner

YIELD: ABOUT 1 CUP
STORAGE: PLASTIC SQUEEZE BOTTLE
TIME: 10 MINUTES

This intensely moisturizing aloe vera and oil blend smoothes split ends by locking in hydration and reversing damaged strands. While fresh aloe vera is preferable in many preparations, this recipe calls for pre-packaged gel to prevent spoilage.

¼ cup coconut oil
½ cup alcohol-free aloe vera gel
¼ cup argan oil
12 drops rosemary essential oil

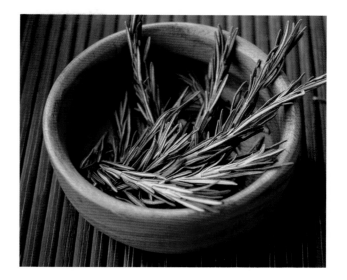

1. In a small saucepan over low heat, warm the coconut oil until melted.
2. Combine the aloe vera gel, argan oil, and coconut oil in a small bowl.
3. Whisk thoroughly to ensure all the moisturizers are thoroughly incorporated.
4. Add the rosemary essential oil and whisk again.
5. Transfer the conditioner to a plastic squeeze bottle. An empty, clean shampoo bottle works well.
6. After washing and conditioning your hair, rinse thoroughly and apply a small amount of this leave-in conditioner to the ends.
7. Dry your hair naturally if possible, then style as usual.
8. Use daily for best results. Keep in the shower.

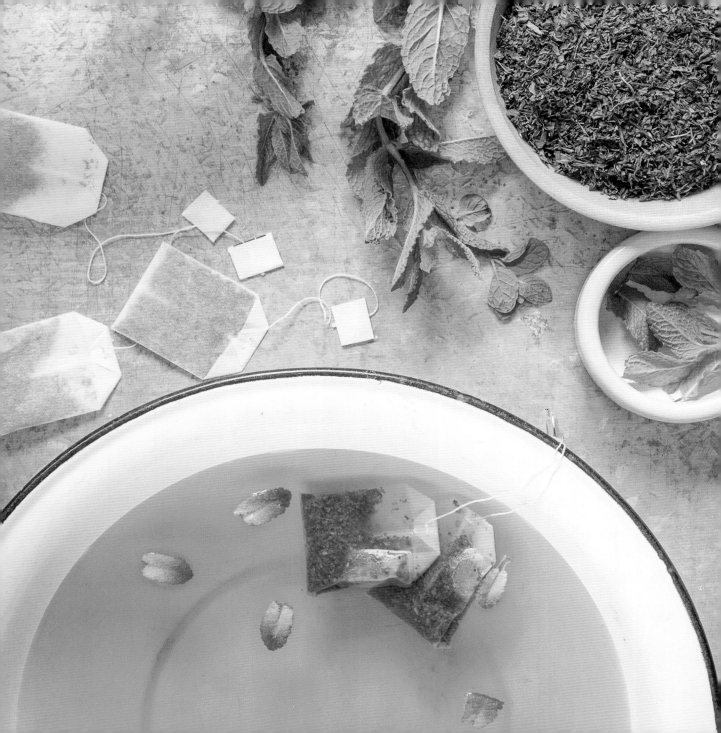

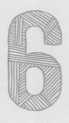

BODY CARE

ATHLETE'S FOOT

Athlete's foot isn't only spread on damp locker room floors anymore. With symptoms including painful blisters, itching, burning, and scaly, cracked skin between the toes, this all-too-common problem is caused by the *tinea* fungus. The good news is that the stronger your immune system, the less likely you are to catch the condition. While there are plenty of over-the-counter treatments, natural remedies can easily do the trick.

Garlic-Tea Tree Foot Soak

YIELD: 1 TREATMENT
STORAGE: NOT RECOMMENDED
TIME: 35 MINUTES

Garlic is one of the best herbs for athlete's foot, particularly when combined with tea tree essential oil. This simple foot soak relieves itching, burning, and redness.

3 cloves garlic, peeled
1 gallon hot water
1 teaspoon rubbing alcohol
2 teaspoons antibacterial liquid soap
10 drops tea tree essential oil

1. In a blender or food processer, purée the garlic into a fine paste.
2. Pour the hot water into a basin or foot bath.
3. Add the rubbing alcohol, antibacterial soap, tea tree essential oil, and garlic.
4. Soak your feet for 30 minutes while sitting comfortably.
5. Towel off, ensuring that your feet are completely dry before putting on socks and shoes.
6. Repeat once daily until your athlete's foot symptoms are gone.

Tea Tree Foot Powder

YIELD: 1 CUP
STORAGE: SUGAR SHAKER
TIME: 5 MINUTES

This one-two punch of baking soda and tea tree oil combines astringents and antifungals to keep feet dry while stopping foot fungus and preventing it from recurring. Use this powder alongside other treatments to maximize its effectiveness.

1 cup baking soda
20 drops tea tree essential oil

1. In a medium bowl, add the baking soda and 5 drops of tea tree essential oil. Blend using a whisk or fork.
2. Add 5 more drops of tea tree essential oil and mix, blending well.
3. Repeat the process until all 20 drops of essential oil have been mixed in.
4. Using a funnel, transfer the foot powder to a sugar shaker.
5. Apply a liberal amount to your socks and shoes before wearing them, and sprinkle on your feet and between your toes after showering.
6. Use once or twice daily. Store in a cool, dry place.

Ginger Foot Balm

YIELD: ABOUT 1 OUNCE
STORAGE: SMALL GLASS JAR
TIME: 24 HOURS

Like garlic, ginger is a strong antifungal herb. This remedy takes some time to prepare, but it leaves your feet with a surprisingly exotic, spicy fragrance. Top with socks at night for smoother skin by morning.

2 tablespoons chopped or finely grated fresh ginger
1 ounce sesame oil

1. In a small jar with a tight-fitting lid, combine the ginger and sesame oil.
2. Place the jar in a warm area for 24 hours.
3. Using a sieve or cheesecloth, strain the oil into a clean jar.
4. Squeeze or press the ginger to extract as much oil as possible.
5. Place a lid on the jar and keep it in the refrigerator between uses.
6. To use, apply a thin layer to affected areas with a cotton ball.
7. Make a new batch if not completely used within 1 week.

❣ Be sure to reapply after showering or bathing, and speed the healing process by applying each night before bed. Continue use for 3 days after the athlete's foot symptoms are gone.

BODY ACNE

Body acne typically responds well to gentle, natural remedies. Harsh chemical antiseptics often cause pain and irritation that can make the affected areas look and feel worse. Whether you've got a mild outbreak on one part of your body or have painful pimples in several places, these simple preparations treat blemishes, improve the condition of the skin, and prevent future spots.

Lavender Bath Salt

YIELD: 1 CUP
STORAGE: GLASS JAR
TIME: 5 MINUTES

Epsom salt is a well-known folk remedy for body acne for good reason. It eases inflammation and helps to purge toxins. Lavender's natural antiseptic properties stop bacteria in its tracks.

1 cup Epsom salt
20 drops lavender essential oil

1. In a medium bowl, add the Epsom salt and 5 drops of lavender essential oil. Blend using a whisk or fork.
2. Add 5 more drops of lavender essential oil and mix, blending well.
3. Repeat the process until all 20 drops of the essential oil have been mixed in.
4. Using a funnel, transfer the bath salt to a glass jar with a tight-fitting lid.
5. To use, mix ¼ cup of the bath salt into a comfortably warm bath.
6. Soak for at least 15 minutes.
7. Use as often as you like. Store in a cool, dry place.

Tea Tree Body Wash

YIELD: ABOUT 1 CUP
STORAGE: PLASTIC SQUEEZE BOTTLE
TIME: 5 MINUTES

Tea tree essential oil is a powerful antibacterial, yet safe for use on blemished skin and effective in easing inflammation and redness. Raw honey smoothes skin texture and fast tracks the healing process.

⅔ cup unscented liquid castile soap
¼ cup raw honey
2 teaspoons sesame oil
1 teaspoon vitamin E oil
60 drops tea tree essential oil

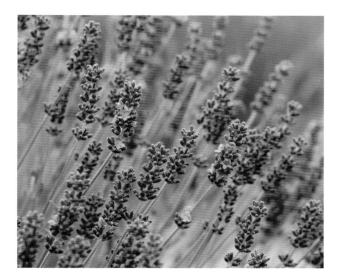

1. In a medium bowl, add the liquid castile soap, raw honey, and sesame oil. Blend using a whisk or fork.
2. Add the vitamin E oil and tea tree essential oil.
3. Blend again, stirring for 30 seconds to ensure all the ingredients are well incorporated.
4. Using a funnel, transfer the body wash to a plastic squeeze bottle. An empty, clean shampoo bottle works well.
5. Squirt a dime-sized amount of body wash onto a bath pouf, washcloth, or bathing brush.
6. Gently scrub your body, paying close attention to the areas where acne is prevalent. Store in a cool, dark place.

BODY ODOR

Body odor isn't exactly the sexiest topic, especially when you're looking for a safe alternative to deodorants with harmful ingredients you can't pronounce. These completely natural, easy-to-prep DIY options take away the riskiness of trial and error (plus the anxiety of going sans protection) because they've been vetted by centuries of proven use.

Lavender–Witch Hazel Freshening Wipes

YIELD: 20 WIPES
STORAGE: GLASS JAR
TIME: 5 MINUTES

Freshen up between showers, post-gym, or before a stressful meeting with handy wipes that kill bacteria in an instant. You can buy a bag of cotton cosmetic pads at your local Walgreens or supermarket for dirt cheap, and you'll use them to make the wipes in this recipe. Both the lavender and witch hazel stop stink fast.

½ cup alcohol-free witch hazel extract
20 drops lavender essential oil
20 cotton cosmetic pads

1. In a glass jar, combine the witch hazel extract and lavender essential oil.
2. Swirl the jar for about 30 seconds to combine the ingredients.
3. Stack the cosmetic pads in the jar.
4. Cap tightly with a lid and shake it gently to ensure all the pads are soaked with the solution.
5. Swab underarms and other smelly areas as needed.

♥ Package a few of these wipes to go by placing them in a plastic storage bag with a secure zip top.

Rosemary Deodorant Bar

YIELD: ABOUT 1½ CUPS
STORAGE: TIN OR PLASTIC STORAGE CONTAINER
TIME: 30 MINUTES

Rosemary and tea tree essential oils stop bacteria production like pros. This fragrant deodorant bar won't stop the sweat, but it will keep you smelling naturally fresh.

3 tablespoons grated beeswax
2 tablespoons coconut oil
1 tablespoon shea butter
2 tablespoons baking soda
2 tablespoons cornstarch
15 drops rosemary essential oil
15 drops tea tree essential oil

1. In a small double boiler, melt the beeswax and coconut oil together.
2. Add the shea butter, stirring constantly until all the ingredients have liquefied.
3. Remove from the heat and pour into a large bowl.
4. Add the baking soda, cornstarch, and rosemary and tea tree essential oils. Blend with a whisk or fork.
5. Working quickly, pour the mixture into a muffin tin, dividing the recipe evenly between two or three cups. ▶

6. Harden at room temperature for 3 hours before use.
7. Rub a small amount of the deodorant onto your underarm area.
8. Apply after your daily bath or shower. Keep in a cool, dry place.

❦ If you happen to have an old deodorant container, you can repurpose it to contain this blend.

CONTACT DERMATITIS

Characterized by itchiness, redness, and perhaps even mild swelling, contact dermatitis occurs when skin is directly exposed to an irritating substance. This can be an immune response to an allergen or the result of minor damage to the skin's delicate upper layer. One thing to watch out for: Because a hot, itchy rash can be a sign of other issues including underlying illness, visit your doctor if symptoms persist or worsen.

Goldenseal Spray

YIELD: 4 OUNCES
STORAGE: SMALL BOTTLE WITH A SPRAY TOP
TIME: 20 MINUTES

This healing spray protects itchy, red skin from further irritation while infusing it with healing herbs. The recipe calls for prepared goldenseal tincture, but feel free to use a goldenseal tincture or infusion you've made at home.

3 ounces purified water
2 teaspoons organic olive oil
1 teaspoon alcohol-free goldenseal tincture

1. Using a funnel, carefully pour the water, olive oil, and goldenseal tincture into a small bottle that can be fitted with a spray top.
2. Screw the top on tightly.
3. Shake well before each use, as the oil will separate from the other ingredients.
4. Spray a light coat of liquid onto the affected area.
5. Apply right after showering, and reapply again before bed for best results. Use as often as needed. Store in a cool, dark place.

Cooling Aloe Vera Gel with Witch Hazel

YIELD: 1 TREATMENT
STORAGE: NOT RECOMMENDED
TIME: 15 MINUTES

This quick gel eases the discomfort of hot, itchy dermatitis faster than it takes to make. For maximum results, take a hot bath or shower right before application to open pores and allow the treatment to penetrate faster.

1 tablespoon alcohol-free aloe vera gel
½ teaspoon alcohol-free witch hazel extract

1. In a small bowl, add the aloe vera gel and the witch hazel extract. Blend with a whisk or fork.
2. Using fingers or a cotton pad, apply the gel to the affected body part and let it penetrate.
3. Wait a few minutes, and then apply a second coat if itching or heat is still present.
4. Reapply every 1 to 2 hours as needed.

❤ Make the treatment more soothing by storing the gel in the refrigerator between uses.

Soothing Calendula Salve with Lavender

YIELD: ABOUT 8 OUNCES
STORAGE: JAR OR TIN
TIME: 10 MINUTES

Make a batch of multipurpose, powerhouse salve as a go-to in your first aid kit. This proven healer is fantastic for treating itchy, irritated skin as well as minor cuts, scrapes, and burns.

7 ounces calendula oil
1 ounce beeswax, grated
½ teaspoon vitamin E oil
10 drops lavender essential oil

1. In a double boiler over low heat, add the calendula oil and beeswax. Blend with a whisk or fork until combined.
2. Remove from the heat as soon as all the beeswax is melted.
3. Add the vitamin E oil and lavender essential oil. Whisk to combine.
4. Pour the salve into a jar or tin.
5. Leave the jar uncovered until the salve cools completely. Once solidified, cover tightly.
6. Apply a thin layer of salve onto the affected area.
7. Use 2 to 3 times daily while recovering from dermatitis. Store in a cool, dark place.

DRY SKIN

It's no secret that dry skin feels itchy, flaky, tight, and uncomfortable, but what you may not know is that herbal remedies are some of the fastest, easiest fixes. Whether your problem is chronic, seasonal, or occasional, you'll find these remedies can be varied to fit almost any lifestyle and severity of condition. While you treat the symptoms, sometimes simple steps like drinking more water, taking cooler showers, and reducing exposure to the elements can nourish dehydrated cells.

Chamomile Milk Bath

YIELD: 1 CUP
STORAGE: AIRTIGHT CONTAINER
TIME: 15 MINUTES

There's a reason milk baths have been used for generations to soften and smooth the body. This particular blend goes one step further by easing itchiness thanks to a concentrated dose of chamomile.

1 cup full-fat powdered milk
24 drops chamomile essential oil

1. Fill the bathtub with warm water.
2. In an airtight container, add the powdered milk and chamomile essential oil and stir to combine.
3. Add 1 cup of milk bath to the bathtub and swish until dissolved.
4. Spend at least 15 minutes soaking in the tub.
5. When you are finished, pat yourself dry. Follow up with your favorite lotion, paying special attention to areas of dry, problem skin.
6. Use once or twice weekly. Store in a cool, dry place.

Geranium Sugar Scrub

YIELD: 6 OUNCES
STORAGE: GLASS JAR OR RESEALABLE PLASTIC CONTAINER
TIME: 5 MINUTES

With geranium, raw honey, and rich almond oil to nourish and moisturize skin, this smoothing scrub also contains sugar to gently exfoliate. If you don't have geranium essential oil, it's not a deal breaker. Try lavender, rosemary, or peppermint instead.

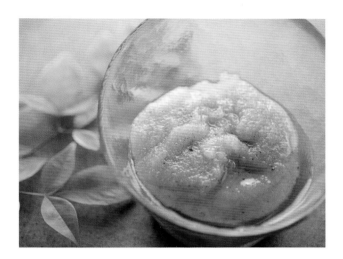

6 tablespoons dark brown sugar

2 ounces almond oil

1 ounce raw honey

6 drops geranium essential oil

1. In a glass jar, add the dark brown sugar, almond oil, and raw honey. Stir gently to combine.
2. Add the geranium essential oil and stir again.
3. Cap tightly with a lid.
4. The almond oil will eventually rise back to the top of the mixture, which is normal. Before showering, mix the sugar scrub with your fingers.
5. Scoop out a tablespoon or so and apply it to your dry skin, rubbing gently while making circular motions.
6. Once you have scrubbed, turn on the water and rinse yourself well, continuing to use light circular motions to buff your skin.
7. When you emerge, pat yourself dry with a soft towel and apply a moisturizer all over. Store in a cool, dry place.

ECZEMA

Eczema is a skin condition often made worse by chemicals found in commercial lotions intended to help symptoms. Herbal remedies will ease the symptoms of eczema—itching, swelling, redness, and flaking—but like commercial lotions, they won't cure the underlying cause, which can be anything from an inherited tendency to allergies, stress, or other lifestyle factors. See your doctor to get to the root issue while using these herbal treatments to give skin TLC.

Burdock Infusion

YIELD: ABOUT 1 CUP
STORAGE: NOT RECOMMENDED
TIME: 15 MINUTES

Burdock tea is one of the most effective natural remedies available for eczema. While the taste leaves something to be desired, you'll get used to it. Adding honey or stevia helps it go down a little easier.

1¼ cups water
1 teaspoon dried burdock root
Raw honey or stevia (optional)

1. In a small saucepan over high heat, combine the water and burdock root. Bring the mixture to a boil.
2. Reduce the heat to medium-low and simmer for 10 minutes.
3. Strain the burdock infusion into a mug, using the back of a spoon to press the liquid from the burdock root before discarding it.
4. Sweeten with raw honey or stevia, if desired.
5. Drink 3 times daily for up to 3 weeks.

Soothing Patchouli Eczema Salve

YIELD: ABOUT 1 CUP
STORAGE: GLASS JAR
TIME: 15 MINUTES

Patchouli grows best in warm climates. Luckily, it's easy to obtain in the form of essential oil. This salve soothes eczema while imparting an intoxicating fragrance.

½ cup coconut oil
8 drops patchouli essential oil
¼ cup oat flour
¼ cup organic olive oil

1. In a small saucepan, melt the coconut oil until it liquefies.
2. Add the patchouli essential oil and the oat flour. Stir until blended.
3. Add the olive oil and mix again, stirring until all the ingredients have been incorporated.
4. Remove from the heat. Pour the salve into a jar and let it cool completely.
5. Cover with a tight cap.
6. Apply a thin layer to the affected area as needed. Keep in a cool, dark place.

♥ This salve has a slightly gritty texture, which is normal. The finely ground oats have healthy fats that help your skin heal.

Comfrey-Plantain Poultice

YIELD: 1 TREATMENT
STORAGE: NOT RECOMMENDED
TIME: 15 MINUTES

Comfrey, plantain leaf, and calendula flowers combine to soothe itching and relieve discomfort quickly. The optional ingredients will make this blend more potent. Apply the poultice as its own treatment or as a complement to other therapies.

1 teaspoon coconut oil, melted
1 teaspoon dried comfrey
1 cup fresh plantain leaves
1 tablespoon fresh calendula flowers or
    1 teaspoon dried calendula flowers
1 tablespoon fresh yarrow leaves or 1 teaspoon dried yarrow leaves (optional)
1 drop rosemary essential oil (optional)

1. In a blender or food processor, combine all ingredients and blend until smooth. If using mostly dried ingredients, you may need to add up to 1 teaspoon of water, a few drops at a time.
2. Using fingertips, apply a thin layer to the affected area.
3. Lay a clean cloth over the herbs, and leave in place for 10 to 15 minutes.
4. Rinse clean with cool water and pat dry.
5. Use 1 to 2 times each day while painful eczema persists.

FOOT ODOR

Notice a foul odor when you kick off your shoes? That's not uncommon. Bacteria are notorious for growing in the dark, moist environment most footwear provides (even your high heels). The trick to kicking the problem is drying up excess moisture **and** adding antibacterial herbs to your foot care regimen to make your skin and shoes less hospitable to odor-causing microbes.

Peppermint Foot Soak

YIELD: 1 TREATMENT
STORAGE: NOT RECOMMENDED
TIME: 20 MINUTES

Peppermint acts as a mild antibacterial while refreshing feet, improving circulation, and imparting a clean, uplifting fragrance.

1 tablespoon dry mint leaves, 3 tablespoons fresh mint leaves, 2 peppermint teabags, or 3 drops peppermint essential oil

1 cup boiling water

1 gallon cool water

1. Add the peppermint to the boiling water and let it steep for 5 minutes.
2. Strain the peppermint from the water (if using fresh or dried leaves).
3. In a shallow basin or footbath, pour the peppermint foot soak into the cool water.
4. Immerse your feet in the basin and relax for 15 minutes.
5. Dry your feet completely, then use a little lotion, foot powder, or foot spray to keep your feet smelling fresh.
6. Use as often as you like.

Quick Tea Tree Foot Spray

YIELD: ABOUT 4 OUNCES
STORAGE: GLASS BOTTLE WITH SPRAY TOP
TIME: 1 MINUTE

With tea tree essential oil to keep bacteria from multiplying, this foot spray imparts a fresh scent that keeps foot odor to a minimum all day.

4 ounces unflavored vodka
12 drops tea tree essential oil

1. In a glass bottle, carefully combine the vodka and the tea tree essential oil.
2. Cap tightly with a spray top.
3. Shake well before each use.
4. Spray all over your feet, ensuring you get between the toes. Wait a few seconds for the spray to dry before putting on socks and shoes.
5. Use daily after bathing or showering. Keep in a cool, dark place.

Lavender-Peppermint Foot Balm

YIELD: 8 OUNCES
STORAGE: GLASS JAR OR TIN
TIME: 20 MINUTES

Pamper tired feet with nourishing moisture and a luxurious fragrance. Spread the love by turning your DIY preparation into a spa gift for anyone who needs a little TLC.

7 ounces organic olive oil
1 ounce beeswax, grated
1 teaspoon vitamin E oil
10 drops lavender essential oil
20 drops peppermint essential oil

1. In a double boiler, add the olive oil and beeswax over low heat. Stir to combine.
2. Remove from the heat once the beeswax melts completely.
3. Stir in the vitamin E oil and the lavender and peppermint essential oils.
4. Transfer to a jar or tin.
5. Cool completely before capping with a tight-fitting lid.
6. Using your fingertips, apply a thin layer to freshly washed feet. Store in a cool, dark place.

For a refreshing at-home spa experience, try the peppermint foot soak and follow up with this balm.

HAND & NAIL CARE

You don't need to book expensive salon appointments to get gorgeous nails. DIY spa treatments contain many of the same natural ingredients you find in high-end products. Plus, make-your-own lets you doctor up the recipes to fit your pampering tastes. Put these remedies in your weekly routine for healthy hands and nails, no manicure required.

Pampering Chamomile-Lavender Scrub

YIELD: 6 OUNCES
STORAGE: GLASS JAR
TIME: 20 MINUTES

If your hands are feeling dry and looking overworked, treat them to a quick pick-me-up. This thick, rich sugar scrub exfoliates and moisturizes, leaving skin feeling refreshed. Try it on dry feet, knees, and elbows too.

6 tablespoons sugar
1 ounce beeswax, grated
2 ounces organic olive oil
4 drops chamomile essential oil
2 drops lavender essential oil

1. Place the sugar in a small jar.
2. In a double boiler over low heat, add the beeswax and olive oil. Stir gently until the beeswax is completely melted.
3. Remove from the heat and cool for 2 minutes.
4. Pour the olive oil and beeswax blend into the jar on top of the sugar, and allow the mixture to cool for 5 minutes.
5. Stir in the chamomile and lavender essential oils and cap the jar tightly.
6. Gently massage your hands with 1 teaspoon of the scrub for at least 1 minute, before rinsing with warm water.
7. Follow up with your favorite moisturizer.
8. Use 3 times weekly for soft, smooth hands. Store in a cook, dark place.

Aloe Vera and Geranium Nail Soak

YIELD: 1 TREATMENT
STORAGE: NOT RECOMMENDED
TIME: 15 MINUTES

With protein-rich gelatin to strengthen nails naturally, this soothing soak also contains aloe vera and geranium for soft, smooth skin.

1 tablespoon unflavored gelatin
½ cup boiling water
1 tablespoon alcohol-free aloe vera gel
4 drops geranium essential oil

1. In a wide bowl, combine the gelatin and water. With a spoon or whisk, stir until the gelatin dissolves completely.
2. Cool until comfortably warm.
3. Stir in the aloe vera gel and geranium essential oil.
4. Immerse your hands into the bowl and let them soak for 5 to 10 minutes.
5. When the water cools, remove your hands and pat them dry with a towel. Follow up with your favorite moisturizer.
6. Repeat once weekly for strong nails that resist cracking and peeling.

Lavender-Sage Hand Salve

YIELD: 8 OUNCES
STORAGE: GLASS JAR OR TIN
TIME: 15 MINUTES

Indulge in this rich salve to comfort and heal dry, cracked skin. Whether your hands are overworked or affected by an arid environment, this soothing remedy brings instant relief.

2 ounces coconut oil
5 ounces organic olive oil
1 ounce beeswax, grated
6 drops lavender essential oil
6 drops sage essential oil

1. In a double boiler, add the coconut oil, olive oil, and beeswax over low heat.
2. When the coconut oil and beeswax melt completely, use a whisk or fork to blend, and remove from the heat.
3. Stir in the lavender and sage essential oils.
4. Transfer to a jar or tin.
5. Cool completely before capping with a tight-fitting lid.
6. Apply a thin layer to clean hands.
7. Use each evening before bed for best results, and apply at other times as needed. Keep in a cool, dark place.

HYPER-PIGMENTATION

Instead of using over-the-counter chemical bleaching agents to deal with hyperpigmentation, why not take care of it naturally? Caused by the over-secretion of natural skin pigment, these dark spots are typically purely cosmetic and can be triggered by sun exposure, hormone imbalance, vitamin and mineral deficiency, and stress. If they're present all over your body, be sure to have your doctor rule out an underlying problem.

Turmeric Facial

YIELD: 1 TREATMENT
STORAGE: NOT RECOMMENDED
TIME: 20 MINUTES

You might know turmeric as one of the spices that gives Indian dishes their signature flavor. This spice also helps to even out skin tone. The downside is that it increases sun sensitivity for a few days after treatment. Be vigilant with sunscreen to prevent burns.

1 teaspoon turmeric
1 teaspoon full-fat powdered milk
3 teaspoons honey

1. In a small dish, add the turmeric, powdered milk, and honey. Using a whisk or fork, stir until blended.
2. With a circular motion, gently scrub your face and other areas affected by hyperpigmentation.
3. After scrubbing, leave the treatment in place for 15 minutes.
4. Rinse your face. Follow up with your favorite cleanser, toner, and moisturizer.
5. Use 3 times weekly until spots have faded.

❧ Because turmeric adheres to the whorls and loops on your fingertips and causes yellowing, it's best to wear disposable latex gloves for this treatment.

Aloe Vera–Lime Mask

YIELD: 1 TREATMENT
STORAGE: NOT RECOMMENDED
TIME: 25 MINUTES

Turns out your grandmother was right: The aloe-vera-and-lime combo does fade dark spots. Together, they lighten excess pigment while sloughing away dead skin and promoting new cell growth.

1 tablespoon alcohol-free aloe vera gel
1 teaspoon fresh lime juice

1. In a small bowl, add the aloe vera gel and lime juice. Using a whisk or fork, mix until smooth.
2. With your fingertips, apply the entire treatment to your freshly washed face.
3. Cover with a paper spa mask and relax for 25 minutes.
4. Repeat 3 times weekly.

Frankincense Facial

YIELD: 1 TREATMENT
STORAGE: NOT RECOMMENDED
TIME: 35 MINUTES

Frankincense essential oil is an excellent weapon in your anti-aging arsenal. The honey and yogurt intensify this treatment, moisturizing while gently exfoliating to renew skin. For pure indulgence, double the dose and apply to hands, neck, and décolletage.

1 teaspoon honey
1 teaspoon yogurt
1 drop frankincense essential oil

1. In a small bowl, add the honey, yogurt, and frankincense essential oil. Using a whisk or fork, blend until smooth.
2. With your fingertips, apply the entire treatment to your face and any other areas with dark spots.
3. Relax for 30 minutes, then rinse with cool water.
4. Follow up with your favorite moisturizer.
5. Repeat 2 to 3 times weekly.

PSORIASIS

Whether caused by an emotional trauma, stress, abnormal liver function, or some other contributing factor, the symptoms—and discomfort—of psoriasis are the same. At its worst, the condition leads to reddish lesions topped by silvery scales of skin that pile up before flaking off, leading to severe itching and bleeding. Use herbal treatments to manage both the skin eruptions and related side effects when psoriasis begins to flare up.

Tea Tree-Licorice Spray

YIELD: ABOUT 8 OUNCES
STORAGE: BOTTLE WITH SPRAY TOP
TIME: 10 MINUTES

With witch hazel extract to stop itching, this spray also contains tea tree, calendula, and licorice to ease pain and promote healing.

1 tablespoon licorice root powder
2 tablespoons calendula oil
7 ounces alcohol-free witch hazel extract
16 drops tea tree essential oil

1. In a medium bowl, add the licorice root powder and calendula oil. Whisk to combine completely.
2. Add 1 ounce of the witch hazel extract and whisk again, stirring until smooth.
3. Add the remainder of the witch hazel extract and stir again.
4. Add the tea tree essential oil and stir again.
5. Using a funnel, transfer the liquid to a bottle with a spray top.
6. Shake well before each use.
7. Spray generously on affected areas.
8. Use at least twice daily while symptoms are present. Store in a cool, dark place.

Goldenseal–St. John's Wort Salve

YIELD: ABOUT 8 OUNCES
STORAGE: GLASS JAR OR TIN
TIME: 15 MINUTES, PLUS 2 WEEKS BREWING

Make this soothing salve ahead of time so you have some on hand when psoriasis flares up. Apply daily during flare-ups to ease pain, swelling, and redness.

1 tablespoon dried goldenseal root
5 ounces organic olive oil
2 ounces coconut oil
1 ounce beeswax, grated
10 drops St. John's wort essential oil
3 drops lavender essential oil
3 drops tea tree essential oil

1. In a glass jar with a tight-fitting lid, combine the dried goldenseal root and the olive oil.
2. Cap the jar tightly and place it in a sunny window for 2 weeks. Every day or two, swirl the jar for 10 seconds.
3. Strain the olive oil into a double boiler. Use the back of a spoon to press as much oil as possible from the root.
4. Add the coconut oil and beeswax to the double boiler.
5. Over low heat, stir gently until the coconut oil and beeswax melt completely.
6. Remove from the heat and cool for 2 minutes.
7. Add the St. John's wort, lavender, and tea tree essential oils and stir again.
8. Carefully transfer to a glass jar or tin. ▶
9. Let the salve cool completely before capping tightly.
10. Using your fingertips, apply a thin layer of salve to affected areas.
11. Repeat 2 to 3 times daily while symptoms are present. Keep in a cool, dark place.

SPIDER VEINS/ VARICOSE VEINS

Appearing as blue and purple lines, usually in the lower legs, spider veins look unsightly and varicose veins often bring aching and throbbing with them. Herbal remedies, support hose, and leg elevation relieve symptoms, but unfortunately don't make the network of veins disappear. See your dermatologist about conventional treatments that can remove them completely.

Lavender–Witch Hazel Spritz

YIELD: ABOUT 8 OUNCES
STORAGE: GLASS BOTTLE WITH SPRAY CAP
TIME: 5 MINUTES

Witch hazel tones and tightens skin, while lavender helps to alleviate pain and inflammation.

1 (8-ounce) bottle alcohol-free witch hazel extract
32 drops lavender essential oil

1. In a glass bottle, combine the witch hazel extract and lavender essential oil.
2. Cap tightly, then shake well.
3. Spray onto your legs each morning and evening, massaging lightly afterward.
4. Use as often as needed to keep your legs feeling comfortable. Store in a cool, dark place between uses.

♥ Package in 3-ounce bottles and stash in your carry-on or gym bag for extra relief during travel or long days on your feet.

Calendula-Chamomile
Leg Liniment

YIELD: ABOUT 8 OUNCES
STORAGE: GLASS BOTTLE
TIME: 5 MINUTES

Calendula and chamomile ease inflammation, while rosemary, lavender, and witch hazel nix discomfort and swelling. Double down on symptoms by massaging the herbs into the skin longer, which increases circulation to the affected areas.

4 ounces alcohol-free witch hazel extract
4 ounces calendula oil
16 drops chamomile essential oil
16 drops lavender essential oil
8 drops rosemary essential oil

1. In a glass bottle, combine all the ingredients.
2. Shake well before each use.
3. With your fingertips, apply about ½ teaspoon of the liniment to each leg. Massage using firm, upward strokes.
4. Use this twice daily. Store in a cool, dark place.

Geranium-Cypress
Massage Blend

YIELD: ABOUT 4 OUNCES
STORAGE: GLASS BOTTLE
TIME: 5 MINUTES

Give legs instant relief with this circulation-enhancing essential oil duo that knocks out pain and discomfort fast. Results are heightened the longer you massage.

4 ounces argan oil
32 drops geranium essential oil
12 drops cypress essential oil

1. In a glass bottle, combine the argan oil with the geranium and cypress essential oils.
2. Cap tightly and shake for 20 seconds to combine.
3. Using your fingertips, apply a thin layer of the blend to the affected areas. Massage using firm, upward strokes.
4. Repeat once or twice daily. Store in a cool, dark place.

SUNBURN

You forgot your sun hat, you didn't apply sunscreen (or reapply after sweating or swimming), or you fell asleep on the beach during prime UV hours. Sunburn happens to the most diligent sun worshipers. Next time you've had too much UV exposure, treat yourself to a quick, simple herbal remedy to ease pain and redness in a flash. The faster you apply these remedies, the lower your chances are of developing blisters and peeling.

Aloe Vera Gel with Lavender

YIELD: 8 OUNCES
STORAGE: PLASTIC SQUEEZE BOTTLE
TIME: 1 MINUTE

Soothe and heal skin with this quick, easy remedy. Keep the bottle in the refrigerator for even more cooling power.

1 (8-ounce) bottle alcohol-free aloe vera gel
32 drops lavender essential oil

1. In a medium bowl, whisk the aloe vera gel and lavender essential oil together.
2. Using a funnel, transfer the gel back into the bottle it came in.
3. Apply liberally after sun exposure, letting the gel penetrate the skin completely before dressing.
4. Reapply at least twice daily while recovering from sunburn.

St. John's Wort Spray with Calendula

YIELD: 8 OUNCES
STORAGE: BOTTLE WITH SPRAY CAP
TIME: 1 MINUTE

This trio is the ultimate first-aid treatment for sunburn. Calendula and St. John's wort ease pain and heal damage, while ultra-cooling witch hazel takes down the temperature of the skin.

7 ounces alcohol-free witch hazel extract
1 ounce calendula oil
16 drops St. John's wort essential oil

1. In a bottle with a spray cap, combine the witch hazel extract, calendula oil, and St. John's wort essential oil.
2. Shake well before each application.
3. Spray liberally on affected areas. Let the witch hazel penetrate the skin completely before dressing.

Keep the bottle in the refrigerator between treatments to maximize its ability to soothe skin.

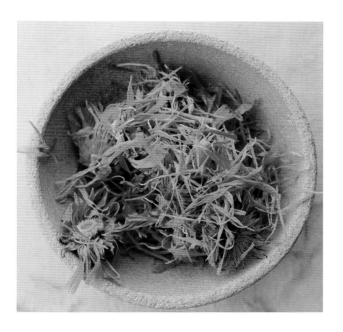

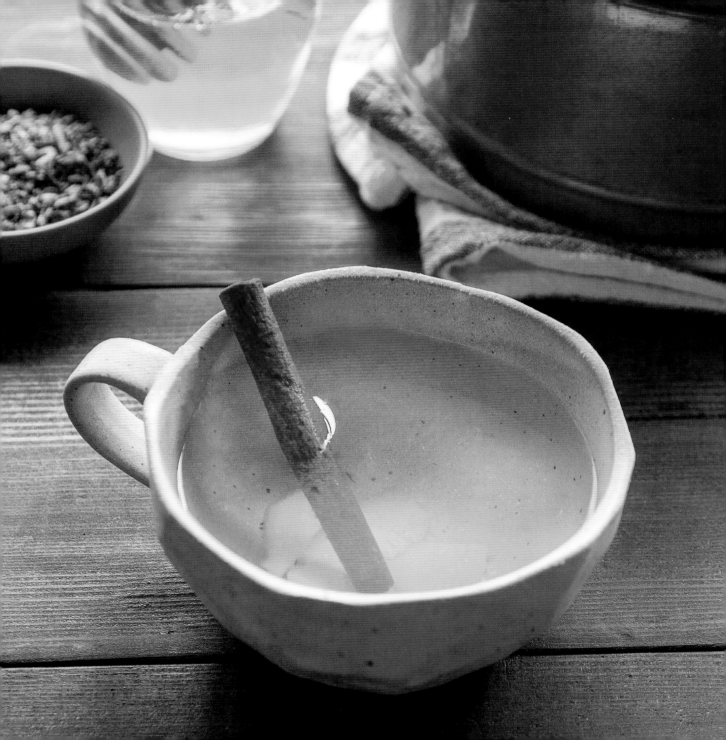

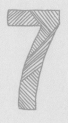

UNDER THE UNDERWEAR

ERECTILE DYSFUNCTION

THE REMEDIES

Also known as ED, erectile dysfunction is exacerbated by smoking, drinking, and lack of physical exercise. If your guy would rather not take prescription drugs with a list of off-putting side effects for a mild case, have him give these herbal remedies a try. Men can, understandably, be sensitive and insecure when it comes to ED. While lifestyle modifications may help too, take things one at a time and exercise as much patience and understanding as you can.

Ginseng Tea

YIELD: 1 CUP
STORAGE: NOT RECOMMENDED
TIME: 15 MINUTES

Most ginseng contains ginsenodes, an ingredient that increases sex drive and stops ED symptoms. Korean ginseng is preferable because it has the most ginsenodes. Don't bother with Siberian ginseng as it's ginsenode-free.

1 tablespoon thinly sliced ginseng root
1 cup boiling water
2 teaspoons raw honey

1. Place the ginseng in a tea ball or infuser. Fill a mug with boiling water and add the tea ball and raw honey.
2. Steep for 15 minutes. Drink.
3. Use twice daily for 3 days, discontinue for 2 weeks, and then use for another 3 days. If the treatment works, continue the cycle for as long as you like.

Saw Palmetto-Pomegranate Juice

YIELD: 8 OUNCES
STORAGE: NOT RECOMMENDED
TIME: 1 MINUTE

You can take saw palmetto supplements daily, but extracts with concentrations of 1:4 or higher may work a bit faster. Drinking pomegranate juice daily may also be helpful.

1 tablespoon saw palmetto extract
8 ounces pomegranate juice
Raw honey or stevia

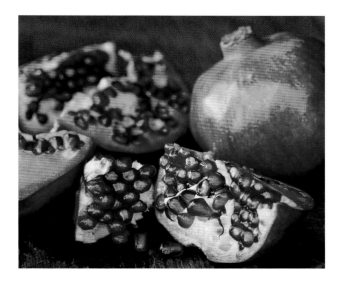

1. In a glass, combine the saw palmetto extract and pomegranate juice.
2. Add ice, if desired.
3. Sweeten with honey or stevia before drinking.
4. Enjoy daily for as long as you like.

JOCK ITCH

Caused by the *trichophyton rubrum* fungus, jock itch can quickly spread throughout the groin area if left untreated. Worse cases can also affect the inner thighs and buttocks. While the herbal treatments for this condition are potent, they work best when you use them as soon as a hot, itchy rash starts to develop. If you experience swelling or pain, see your doctor to rule out a more serious condition.

Witch Hazel–Tea Tree Antifungal Spray

YIELD: 8 OUNCES
STORAGE: GLASS BOTTLE WITH SPRAY TOP
TIME: 5 MINUTES

This remedy eases discomfort by relieving itchiness while providing a pleasant, cooling sensation. The tea tree essential oil kills the fungus that causes jock itch.

1 (8-ounce) bottle alcohol-free witch hazel extract
80 drops tea tree essential oil

1. In a glass bottle, combine the witch hazel extract and tea tree essential oil.
2. Shake well before each use.
3. Spray the affected area with a thin coat of liquid after showering and toweling off.
4. Let the remedy penetrate before dressing.
5. Apply at least twice daily for best results, and keep using for 3 days after symptoms disappear to be certain that the fungus is gone for good. Store in a cool, dark place.

Garlic Salve

YIELD: 1 TREATMENT
STORAGE: NOT RECOMMENDED
TIME: 5 MINUTES

Garlic is a powerful antifungal agent that helps stop jock itch quickly. While you might be tempted to make a big batch of this remedy to save some time, freshly ground garlic works best.

5 cloves fresh garlic, peeled
1 teaspoon organic olive oil

1. In a blender or food processer, combine the garlic and olive oil.
2. Using a fine strainer over a small bowl, separate the pulp from the garlic juice and oil.
3. Apply to the affected area with a cotton ball, working from the outside of the rash toward its center.
4. Use twice daily for best results, and keep using for 3 days after symptoms disappear to be certain that the fungus is gone for good.

Ginger-Thyme Wash

YIELD: APPROXIMATELY 10 TREATMENTS
STORAGE: REFRIGERATE IN GLASS BOTTLE OR JAR
TIME: 25 MINUTES

Ginger and thyme ease itching and redness while killing the fungi that cause jock itch. This remedy is a good one to use for ringworm and athlete's foot, too.

1 cup boiling water
1 tablespoon peeled, finely grated fresh ginger root
1 tablespoon dried thyme leaves or 2 tablespoons fresh thyme leaves

1. In a small bowl, combine all the ingredients.
2. Allow the mixture to steep for 20 minutes. Once cool, transfer it to a glass bottle or jar with a tight-fitting lid.
3. To prevent contamination, pour a small amount into a separate container before use.
4. With a cotton pad, apply a generous amount to the affected area.
5. Allow to air dry.
6. Repeat 1 to 2 times each day while jock itch symptoms persist. The wash will remain fresh, when refrigerated, for up to a week.

MENSTRUAL PAIN & CRAMPS

Ranging from mildly annoying to unbearable, menstrual pain and cramps typically begin at the same time as your period and continue for 2 to 3 days. These remedies relax muscles, ease contractions, and lessen discomfort. Contact your doctor if you develop a fever with cramping, or if your symptoms are occurring outside the normal time frame. Fibroids, abnormal pregnancies, ovarian cysts, and other potentially dangerous conditions cause similar symptoms.

Black Cohosh Tea

YIELD: 1 CUP
STORAGE: NOT RECOMMENDED
TIME: 15 MINUTES

This tea is a traditional remedy for pain and cramping associated with menstruation thanks to an effective roundup of anti-inflammatories and pain relievers. Black cohosh, the least well-known ingredient, contains salicylic acid, which has the same inflammation-reducing effects as aspirin.

1 cup water
1 teaspoon dried black cohosh
¼ teaspoon powdered cinnamon
¼ teaspoon powdered ginger
Honey or stevia (optional)

1. In a small saucepan, bring the water to a boil. Remove from the heat, and add the black cohosh, cinnamon, and ginger.
2. Steep for 15 minutes, then strain the tea through cheesecloth into a mug.
3. Sweeten with honey or stevia, if desired, and drink while relaxing.
4. Drink 3 to 4 cups daily when pain and cramps are a problem.

Raspberry-Lemon Balm Tea

YIELD: 1 CUP
STORAGE: NOT RECOMMENDED
TIME: 15 MINUTES

Ease pain and cramping with this miraculous lineup of muscle relaxers. The beauty of this recipe is that you don't need all five herbs to alleviate symptoms. Missing one or two? Replace them with a little bit more of the ones you do have.

- **1 cup water**
- **1 teaspoon dried catnip**
- **1 teaspoon dried clary sage**
- **1 teaspoon dried lemon balm**
- **1 teaspoon dried raspberry leaf**
- **¼ teaspoon dried ginger**
- **Honey or stevia (optional)**

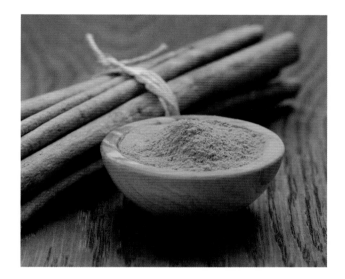

1. In a small saucepan, bring the water to a boil. Add the herbs and remove from the heat.
2. Steep for 15 minutes, then strain the tea through cheesecloth into a mug, using the back of a spoon to press the excess liquid from the herbs.
3. Sweeten with honey or stevia, if desired, and drink while relaxing.
4. Drink 3 to 4 cups of this tea each day while pain and cramps are present.

PAINFUL SEX

If vaginal dryness is causing discomfort during sex, try one of these natural lubricants instead of a pricey commercial one made with some of the same chemicals found in products like brake fluid and oven cleaner. In the meantime, work with your doctor to determine whether the underlying cause is a more serious gynecological condition.

Ylang-Ylang Lubricating Balm

YIELD: 8 OUNCES
STORAGE: GLASS JAR OR TIN
TIME: 15 MINUTES

With coconut oil that changes from solid to liquid when warmed, this lubricant contains ylang-ylang essential oil, which also acts as a natural aphrodisiac.

8 ounces coconut oil
½ teaspoon ylang-ylang essential oil

1. In a double boiler, melt the coconut oil over low heat.
2. Remove from the heat when liquefied and cool for 2 minutes.
3. Add the ylang-ylang essential oil and stir to combine.
4. Pour the balm into a glass jar or tin.
5. Cool completely before capping tightly.
6. Using your fingertips, apply to intimate areas before sex. Use as much as is needed.
7. This lubricant is safe to use as often as you like. Store it in a cool, dark place.

Warming Geranium-Jasmine Lubricating Balm

YIELD: 4 OUNCES
STORAGE: GLASS BOTTLE
TIME: 15 MINUTES

With nourishing almond oil to lubricate, plus geranium and jasmine essential oils to help balance your hormones, this balm contains peppermint essential oil for a warm, tingly sensation.

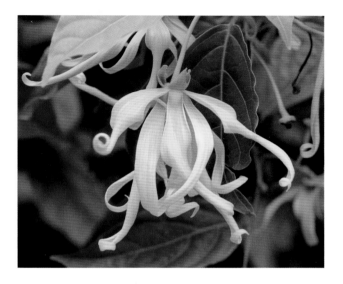

- **4 ounces almond oil**
- **10 drops geranium essential oil**
- **10 drops jasmine essential oil**
- **3 drops peppermint essential oil**

1. In a glass bottle, combine all the ingredients.
2. Shake well to blend.
3. Shake for 2 to 3 seconds before each use.
4. Apply a small amount to intimate areas before sex. Use as much as is needed.
5. This lubricant is safe to use as often as you like. Store in a cool, dark place.

❤ Omit the peppermint if you prefer to use lubricant that doesn't tingle.

URINARY TRACT INFECTION

THE REMEDIES

Urinary tract infections (UTIs) occur when bacteria multiplies in the urethral opening and travels up toward the bladder. Start using natural remedies as soon as you notice pain or an urgent need to urinate even though your bladder is already empty. If you develop a fever or symptoms fail to improve within two days, see your doctor for antibiotics.

Cranberry-Green Tea Tonic

YIELD: ½ GALLON
STORAGE: REFRIGERATE IN PITCHER
TIME: 15 MINUTES

Put a traditional cranberry UTI remedy into overdrive by pairing it with green tea. The combination reduces bladder inflammation and kills the infection-causing bacteria more effectively than fighting with cranberry alone.

4 cups boiling water
4 green tea bags
4 cups unsweetened cranberry juice
Honey or stevia (optional)

1. In a saucepan, combine the boiling water and green tea bags.
2. Steep for 15 minutes, then discard the tea bags.
3. In a pitcher, combine the green tea, cranberry juice, and honey or stevia, if desired.
4. Drink the entire pitcher of tea and juice over the course of the day.
5. Repeat each day while fighting a urinary tract infection.

Saw Palmetto Tea

YIELD: 1 CUP
STORAGE: NOT RECOMMENDED
TIME: 5 MINUTES

Like cranberries, saw palmetto berries are useful in treating urinary tract infections. Of all types of saw palmetto supplements available, extract provides relief fastest. Find it at a health food store or online.

1 tablespoon saw palmetto extract
1 cup hot water
Honey or stevia (optional)

1. In a mug, combine the saw palmetto extract, hot water, and honey or stevia, if desired, and drink.
2. Take twice daily for up to 3 days.

♥ Saw palmetto extract has a slightly acidic taste. If you dislike the tea, blend the extract with about a tablespoon of cool water and drink it all at once.

Mullein Tea

YIELD: 1 CUP
STORAGE: NOT RECOMMENDED
TIME: 15 MINUTES

Mullein leaf has a soothing effect on the urinary tract. In addition, it acts as a mild diuretic that promotes urination, helping to flush bacteria from your bladder.

2 teaspoons crumbled dried mullein leaf
1 cup boiling water

1. Put the mullein leaf in a tea ball or infuser, and place in a mug of boiling water.
2. Steep for 15 minutes. Drink.
3. Enjoy 2 to 3 cups daily for up to 3 days.

♥ Mullein is a mild sedative. Do not drink this tea before driving or doing other tasks that require concentration.

VAGINAL ODOR

True, vaginal odor is an embarrassing issue, but the good news is that it also serves as an indicator that the beneficial bacteria—a.k.a. *Lactobacilli*—inhabiting your nether region is out of balance. If you've been taking antibiotics, cleansing with commercial feminine hygiene products, or using douches frequently (all of which deplete the vagina's healthy bacteria population), use these preparations to bring your vaginal flora back into balance.

Lavender Suppository

YIELD: 1 TREATMENT
STORAGE: NOT RECOMMENDED
TIME: 30 MINUTES

Plain yogurt with live, active cultures contains Lactobacillus bacteria, and lavender essential oil helps to kill off fungus that could be contributing to the unpleasant odor.

1 tablespoon plain yogurt
2 drops lavender essential oil

1. In a small bowl, combine the yogurt and lavender essential oil.
2. Apply the entire amount to a tampon. If using a tampon with an applicator, remove the cotton portion and coat it with the yogurt mixture.
3. Insert the suppository into your vagina. Remove and discard it after 30 minutes.
4. Repeat the treatment twice daily for 3 days in a row.

Cleansing Tea Tree Bath

YIELD: 1 TREATMENT
STORAGE: NOT RECOMMENDED
TIME: 30 MINUTES

Tea tree essential oil, baking soda, and apple cider vinegar combine to eliminate excess bacteria. If you have no tea tree essential oil, try lavender or eucalyptus instead.

2 cups apple cider vinegar
6 drops tea tree essential oil
½ cup baking soda

1. Draw a warm bath.
2. Add the apple cider vinegar and tea tree essential oil to the bath, then swish with your hand.
3. Sprinkle the baking soda on top of the water.
4. Soak in the tub for 30 minutes, opening your legs to let the water make full contact with the exterior portion of your vagina.
5. After bathing, dry your body well. Excess moisture feeds the bacteria that lead to vaginal odor.
6. Use this treatment once daily for as long as needed. Keep your vaginal area dry by wearing cotton underwear and using body powder before dressing each day.

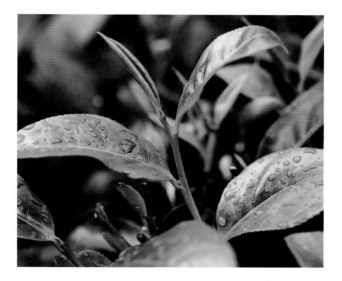

YEAST INFECTION

If you've ever had a yeast infection, you're probably all too familiar with the accompanying itchiness, soreness, and smelly white discharge. Usually caused by a fungus called *Candida albicans,* yeast infections thrive on sugars that are delivered via the bloodstream. Shorten their duration by cutting back on sugar while giving these natural remedies a chance to work. Eating garlic and taking probiotics can help, too.

Garlic Suppository

YIELD: 1 TREATMENT
STORAGE: NOT RECOMMENDED
TIME: OVERNIGHT

Put garlic up there? Um, yes. This truly alternative remedy is one that works best during the beginning stage of a yeast infection when the herb's antibacterial forces can get to work. Use it as soon as you notice itching.

1 clove fresh garlic, peeled

1. Wrap a clove of garlic in a piece of gauze.
2. Encase the garlic by tying the open end of the gauze securely with a piece of thread. Leave 3 to 4 inches of thread hanging from the suppository.
3. Insert the suppository into your vagina at bedtime. Remove and discard it in the morning.
4. Repeat the treatment for 3 to 5 nights in a row. If symptoms worsen or fail to improve, see your doctor for something stronger.

Tea Tree Douche

YIELD: 1 TREATMENT
STORAGE: NOT RECOMMENDED
TIME: 10 MINUTES

Tea tree essential oil and apple cider vinegar work in tandem to greatly reduce the vagina's yeast population. Use this treatment as soon as you notice symptoms. This remedy requires the purchase of a douche—a rubber bulb with a smoothed, curved nozzle—that you can find online.

2 quarts warm distilled water
3 tablespoons apple cider vinegar
2 drops tea tree essential oil

1. In a pitcher or large jar, combine all the ingredients.
2. Transfer to a douche and use per the manufacturer's instructions.
3. Repeat twice daily for up to 5 days, until symptoms are gone. If symptoms worsen or fail to improve, see your doctor for something stronger.

Lavender-Myrrh Bath

YIELD: 1 TREATMENT
STORAGE: NOT RECOMMENDED
TIME: 20 MINUTES

Lavender, myrrh, and tea tree essential oils are potent antifungal agents, and coconut oil contains fatty acids that work against yeast. This bath helps to relieve discomfort while imparting aromatherapy benefits. Just relaxing for a while can help you feel better and, as an added benefit, your skin will feel soft and smooth when you emerge from the bath.

1 tablespoon coconut oil
10 drops lavender essential oil
6 drops myrrh essential oil
4 drops tea tree essential oil

1. Draw a warm bath.
2. Add the coconut oil and essential oils.
3. Spend 15 to 20 minutes in the bath with the lower half of your body fully submerged.
4. After getting out of the bath, thoroughly dry your body, and especially the genital area.
5. Enjoy this bath treatment 1 to 2 times each day while the infection persists. It is an excellent complement to other treatments.

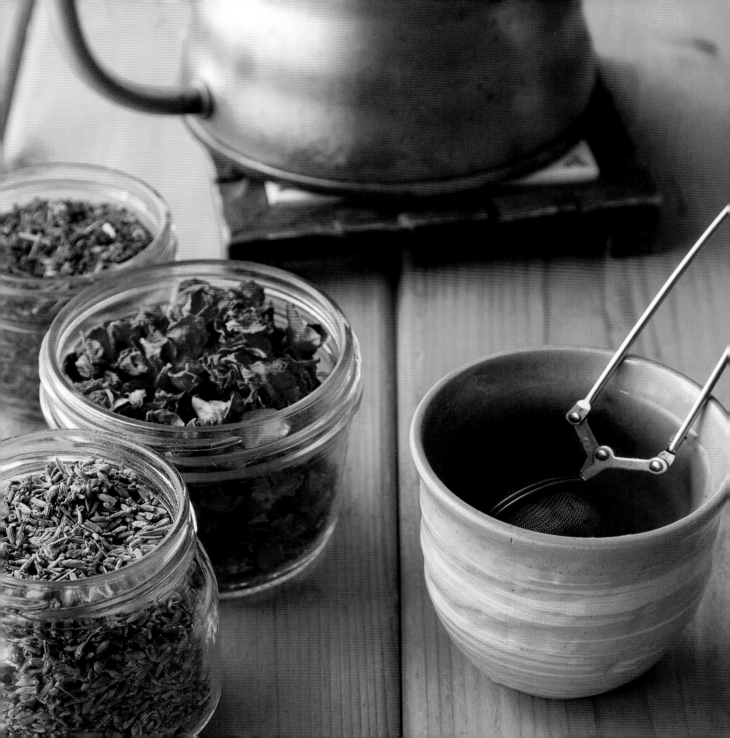

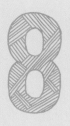

MENTAL HEALTH AND WELLNESS

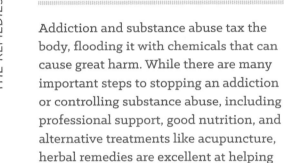

ADDICTION & SUBSTANCE ABUSE

Addiction and substance abuse tax the body, flooding it with chemicals that can cause great harm. While there are many important steps to stopping an addiction or controlling substance abuse, including professional support, good nutrition, and alternative treatments like acupuncture, herbal remedies are excellent at helping you manage tough withdrawal symptoms.

St. John's Wort–Lemon Balm Tea Blend

YIELD: 2½ CUPS
STORAGE: AIRTIGHT CONTAINER
TIME: 5 MINUTES

Sometimes referred to as "nature's Prozac," St. John's wort boosts your brain's serotonin levels, lifting your mood and bringing some relief from the effects of withdrawal. The lemon balm imparts an uplifting fragrance.

1½ cups dried St. John's wort
1 cup dried lemon balm leaves
1 cup boiling water
Honey or stevia (optional)

1. In an airtight container, combine the St. John's wort and lemon balm leaves.
2. Add 1 teaspoon of the herb mixture to a tea ball or infuser, and place in a mug of boiling water.
3. Steep for 10 to 15 minutes.
4. Add some honey or stevia to sweeten, if desired.
5. Drink 2 cups of this tea each day.

❤ St. John's wort works best when taken regularly, and it can take between 2 and 3 weeks for you to really notice its effects.

Milk Thistle Liver Cleanse

YIELD: 1 TREATMENT
STORAGE: NOT RECOMMENDED
TIME: 5 MINUTES

Enjoy this cleanse as part of a complete detox. Milk thistle contains sylmarin, a combination of three powerful antioxidants that protect and repair liver cells while reducing inflammation.

20 drops milk thistle extract
1 teabag, any flavor
1 cup boiling water

1. In a mug, combine the milk thistle extract, teabag, and boiling water.
2. Steep for 5 minutes.
3. Sweeten, if desired. Drink 4 cups per day before meals and snacks.
4. Use this remedy for 1 to 2 weeks while detoxifying your body.

Dandelion Tonic

YIELD: 1 CUP
STORAGE: NOT RECOMMENDED
TIME: 10 MINUTES

Help your liver, kidneys, and spleen heal while clearing toxins with this simple tonic. Its taste is smooth, mellow, and mild, and drinking it will help you feel better.

2 teaspoons chopped dandelion root
1½ cups water
2 teaspoons raw honey

1. In a small saucepan, combine the dandelion root, water, and raw honey. Bring to a boil.
2. Reduce the heat to medium-low and simmer for 15 minutes.
3. Pour into a mug and cool slightly.
4. Drink 2 cups of tonic daily while recovering from substance abuse.

ADHD

Characterized by impulsivity, hyperactivity, and inattention, attention deficit hyperactivity disorder (ADHD) commonly affects children but often lasts into or starts in adulthood. Conventional prescriptive medications used to treat ADHD are stimulants. Like these drugs, stimulant herbs can have a calming effect, diminishing symptoms and enhancing focus. Never stop taking prescriptions for ADHD without first consulting your doctor.

Ginkgo Biloba Tea

YIELD: ABOUT 1 CUP
STORAGE: NOT RECOMMENDED
TIME: 15 MINUTES

Ginkgo biloba helps increase focus, and it also helps enhance your memory. If you take prescriptions of any kind, be sure to speak to your doctor before use.

1 tablespoon crushed dried ginkgo biloba
1¼ cups boiling water
Honey or stevia (optional)

1. Place the ginkgo in a tea ball or infuser. In a mug filled with boiling water, add the tea ball.
2. Steep for 15 minutes.
3. Add honey or stevia to sweeten, if desired, and drink.
4. Enjoy this tea once or twice daily during the morning and early afternoon hours.

Ginseng-Spice Iced Tea

YIELD: ½ GALLON
STORAGE: REFRIGERATE IN PITCHER
TIME: 30 MINUTES

Ginseng can boost dopamine levels, help you focus, and improve your memory. Use American or Korean ginseng, as they are more effective than Siberian ginseng. Sweet spices add flavor.

8 tablespoons chopped dried ginseng root
2 whole cinnamon sticks
5 whole cloves
1 tablespoon peeled, grated fresh ginger root
8 cups water
Honey or stevia (optional)

1. In a saucepan, combine the ginseng root, cinnamon, cloves, ginger, and water. Bring to a boil.
2. Remove from the heat. Let the herbs steep for 15 minutes.
3. Strain the tea into a pitcher, using the back of a spoon to press the excess liquid from the herbs.
4. Cool to room temperature.
5. Sweeten with honey or stevia, if desired. Serve over ice.
6. Store in the refrigerator.
7. Drink 2 to 4 glasses of tea daily, during the morning and early afternoon hours. Cut back if you have trouble sleeping.

Lavender Smelling Salt

YIELD: 1 OUNCE
STORAGE: SMALL GLASS JAR
TIME: 2 MINUTES

Lavender essential oil stimulates the limbic system, helping you to manage your emotions and form new memories. It also aids focus while helping you feel calm and relaxed.

1 ounce coarse sea salt
20 drops lavender essential oil

1. In a small jar, combine the sea salt and lavender essential oil.
2. Cap tightly and shake well to blend.
3. Inhale deeply for 20 seconds.
4. Use as needed to increase focus. Refresh with more lavender essential oil when the fragrance begins to fade.

ANXIETY—OCD

Natural remedies for obsessive-compulsive disorder (OCD) help stop nervousness while promoting relaxation and heightening focus. The herbs used in these treatments are well known for their ability to alleviate the stress that leads to anxiety, either when used alone or alongside conventional treatments. If you're taking any prescriptions, talk to your doctor before using herbal remedies.

Bergamot Smelling Salt

YIELD: 1 OUNCE
STORAGE: SMALL GLASS JAR
TIME: 2 MINUTES

Bergamot calms nervousness, focuses the thoughts, and helps eliminate stressful feelings. This smelling salt can help improve your state of mind quickly.

1 ounce coarse sea salt
20 drops bergamot essential oil

1. In a small glass jar, combine the sea salt with the bergamot essential oil.
2. Cap tightly and shake well to blend.
3. Inhale deeply for 20 seconds.
4. Use this remedy as often as you like to ease anxiety and refocus your mind. Refresh the salt with additional essential oil when the fragrance begins to fade.

Chamomile-Ginger Tea with Licorice

YIELD: 1 CUP
STORAGE: NOT RECOMMENDED
TIME: 15 MINUTES

When focus and calm are what you need, look to chamomile, ginger, and licorice to keep nervousness and racing thoughts at bay. Its sweet, spicy taste makes it a delicious option as an everyday drink.

1 tablespoon dried chamomile flowers
1 teaspoon peeled, grated fresh ginger root
1 teaspoon chopped dried licorice root
1¼ cups water

1. In a small saucepan, combine the chamomile, ginger, licorice, and water. Bring to a boil.
2. Reduce the heat to medium-low and simmer for 15 minutes.
3. Strain the tea into a mug, using the back of a spoon to press the excess liquid from the herbs before discarding them.
4. Drink the tea anytime you are feeling anxious. Enjoy it as often as you like.

St. John's Wort-Passionflower Tonic

YIELD: 1 CUP
STORAGE: NOT RECOMMENDED
TIME: 15 MINUTES

St. John's wort and passionflower combine to help ease frayed nerves while reducing anxiety and calming the mind. This relaxing blend is best enjoyed when you have time to unwind.

1 tablespoon dried St. John's wort
1 tablespoon dried passionflower
1 cup boiling water

1. In a mug, combine the St. John's wort, passionflower, and boiling water.
2. Steep for 15 minutes.
3. Drink each night before bed. Do not use before driving or doing other tasks that require you to concentrate.

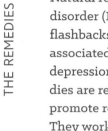

ANXIETY– PTSD

Natural remedies for post-traumatic stress disorder (PTSD) can help relieve terrifying flashbacks and nightmares, along with associated problems like insomnia and depression. The herbs used in these remedies are renowned for their ability to promote relaxation while alleviating stress. They work best when taken in conjunction with conventional treatments such as talk therapy. If you're taking medications, talk to your doctor before adding herbal treatments or stopping prescriptions.

Hyssop–Peppermint Tea

YIELD: 1 CUP
STORAGE: NOT RECOMMENDED
TIME: 15 MINUTES

When hyssop and peppermint team up, nerves and stress don't last long. This fragrant blend also happens to be a secret weapon against cold and flu symptoms.

1 teaspoon crumbled dried hyssop leaves
1 teaspoon crumbled dried peppermint leaves
1 cup boiling water
Honey or stevia (optional)

1. Place the hyssop and peppermint leaves in a tea ball or infuser. In a mug filled with boiling water, add the tea ball, and honey or stevia, if desired.
2. Steep for 15 minutes.
3. Drink hot or iced as often as you like.

Lavender-St. John's Wort Smelling Salt

YIELD: 1 OUNCE
STORAGE: SMALL GLASS JAR
TIME: 2 MINUTES

When anxiety has got you down, lavender and St. John's wort can lift your spirits back up. This ultra-relaxing blend also brings calm and focus when your thoughts are racing.

1 ounce coarse sea salt
20 drops lavender essential oil
2 drops St. John's wort essential oil

1. In a small glass jar, combine the salt and lavender and St. John's wort essential oils.
2. Cap tightly and shake well to blend.
3. Inhale deeply for 20 seconds.
4. Use this blend as often as you like. Refresh it with more essential oil when the fragrance begins to fade.

Valerian Infusion

YIELD: 1 CUP
STORAGE: NOT RECOMMENDED
TIME: 15 MINUTES

Valerian helps ease anxiety while promoting deep relaxation. This tea is powerful, so enjoy it when you have time to unwind.

1 teaspoon crumbled dried peppermint
1 teaspoon dried chopped valerian root
1¼ cups water
Raw honey or stevia (optional)

1. In a small saucepan, combine the peppermint, valerian root, and water.
2. Bring to a boil.
3. Reduce the heat to medium-low and allow the herbs to simmer for 10 minutes.
4. Remove from the heat and strain into a mug.
5. Sweeten with raw honey or stevia, if desired.
6. Drink while relaxing. Do not use before driving or undertaking other tasks that require high levels of concentration.

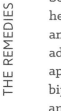

BIPOLAR DISORDER

Some herbal remedies for bipolar disorder help manage symptoms such as irritability, anxiety, and impulsive behavior. Others address depressive symptoms, like poor appetite and low mood. The seriousness of bipolar disorder cannot be overstated, and an herbal approach should not be the sole approach to managing it. Do not discontinue prescriptions or supplement with herbal remedies without consulting your doctor in case of potential harmful drug interactions.

Mandarin-Peppermint Smelling Salt

YIELD: 1 OUNCE
STORAGE: SMALL GLASS JAR
TIME: 2 MINUTES

Mandarin and peppermint combine to alleviate depressive symptoms. This smelling salt can be used alongside other therapies if needed.

1 ounce coarse sea salt
20 drops mandarin essential oil
10 drops peppermint essential oil

1. In a small glass jar, combine the salt and the mandarin and peppermint essential oils.
2. Cap tightly and shake well to blend.
3. Inhale deeply for 20 seconds.
4. Enjoy this remedy as often as you like. Refresh the blend with more essential oil when the fragrance begins to fade.

Lavender Linen Spray

YIELD: 8 OUNCES
STORAGE: GLASS BOTTLE WITH A SPRAY TOP
TIME: 5 MINUTES

Lavender essential oil calms nervousness and helps stop racing thoughts. This linen spray smells wonderful and makes your bed a more relaxing place to be.

8 ounces water
1 teaspoon lavender essential oil

1. In a glass bottle, combine the water with the lavender essential oil.
2. Shake tightly before each use.
3. Just before bed, spray your sheets and pillows with the linen spray.
4. Use nightly. Inhale deeply while relaxing as you fall asleep.

Herbal Balancing Tea

YIELD: ABOUT 1 CUP
STORAGE: NOT RECOMMENDED
TIME: 15 MINUTES

Chamomile, hyssop, rosemary, and mint combine to alleviate stress and promote a balanced mood. Inhale the steam while the herbs steep. The fragrance will help you feel slightly relaxed.

1¼ cups water
1 tablespoon dried chamomile flowers
1 teaspoon crushed dried hyssop
1 teaspoon crushed dried mint
½ teaspoon crushed dried rosemary
Honey or stevia (optional)

1. In a small saucepan, boil the water. Add the chamomile, hyssop, mint, and rosemary. Remove from the heat.
2. Steep for 15 minutes.
3. Strain into a mug, pressing excess liquid from the herbs before discarding them.
4. Sweeten with honey or stevia, if desired, and drink.
5. Enjoy this tea as often as you like.

DEPRESSION

Mild depression impacts your mood, making it difficult, and many days impossible, for you to enjoy daily activities. Herbal remedies can lift your spirits and sharpen your thinking while helping to increase your interest in the things that are important to you. They can also help you stay alert during the day and sleep better at night. If these remedies don't help, talk to your doctor about other treatment options.

Uplifting St. John's Wort Smelling Salt

YIELD: 1 OUNCE
STORAGE: SMALL GLASS JAR
TIME: 2 MINUTES

St. John's wort, lavender, and rosemary combine to ease feelings of mild depression. This smelling salt can be used alongside other treatments.

1 ounce coarse sea salt
10 drops lavender essential oil
10 drops rosemary essential oil
10 drops St. John's wort essential oil

1. In a small jar, combine the salt and the lavender, rosemary, and St. John's wort essential oils.
2. Cap tightly and shake well to blend.
3. Inhale deeply for 20 seconds.
4. Use this remedy as often as you like. Refresh the blend with additional essential oil when the fragrance begins to fade.

Spiced Licorice-Lemon Balm Infusion

YIELD: ABOUT 1 CUP
STORAGE: NOT RECOMMENDED
TIME: 15 MINUTES

Licorice, cloves, and lemon balm work together to lift feelings of minor depression. You can replace the lemon balm with peppermint if you like.

1 teaspoon chopped dried licorice root
1 tablespoon crushed dried lemon balm
3 whole cloves
1¼ cups water
Honey or stevia (optional)

1. In a small saucepan, add the licorice, lemon balm, and cloves to the water. Bring to a boil.
2. Reduce the heat to medium-low and simmer for 10 minutes.
3. Strain into a mug, using the back of a spoon to press the excess liquid from the herbs before discarding them.
4. Sweeten with honey or stevia, if desired.
5. Enjoy a cup of this comforting tea anytime you need a mental lift.

Feel Good Herbal Tea Blend

YIELD: 4 CUPS DRIED HERBAL BLEND
STORAGE: AIRTIGHT CONTAINER
TIME: 15 MINUTES

This herbal blend brings fast relief from feelings of minor depression. If you take antidepressants, either omit the St. John's wort or talk to your doctor about including it in your daily regimen.

1½ cups crushed dried lemon balm
½ cup dried lavender
½ cup dried marjoram
½ cup dried rose petals
½ cup crushed dried spearmint
½ cup dried St. John's wort
1 cup boiling water
Vanilla, lemon, or honey (optional)

1. In an airtight container, combine all the herbs.
2. To brew the tea, use 1 tablespoon of the herbal blend per cup, and place in a tea ball or infuser.
3. In a mug, pour boiling water over the herbs and steep for 15 minutes.
4. Flavor with vanilla, lemon, or honey, if desired.
5. Drink up to 3 cups of tea daily to alleviate minor depression.

EATING DISORDERS

An eating disorder—whether it causes you to undereat, overeat, or binge and purge—can take over your life. These herbal remedies are best when used alongside conventional treatments such as talk therapy. They aid in supporting the healthy lifestyle changes you want to make, as well as balance hormones and manage triggers like stress.

Licorice-Ginseng Tonic

YIELD: ABOUT 1 CUP
STORAGE: NOT RECOMMENDED
TIME: 15 MINUTES

Ease bulimia symptoms with this tonic. The licorice helps to stabilize blood sugar while the ginseng relieves stress. Together, they reduce the desire to overeat.

1 tablespoon chopped dried licorice root
1 teaspoon chopped ginseng root
1¼ cups water

1. In a small saucepan, add the licorice and ginseng to the water. Bring to a boil.
2. Reduce the heat to medium-low and simmer the herbs for 10 minutes.
3. Strain into a mug, using the back of a spoon to press excess liquid from the herbs before discarding them.
4. Drink a cup of this tonic 2 to 3 times daily, especially when the urge to binge arises.

Lemon Balm-Yarrow Tea

YIELD: 1 CUP
STORAGE: NOT RECOMMENDED
TIME: 15 MINUTES

Lemon balm and yarrow combine to stimulate appetite, helping to encourage sufferers of anorexia to eat.

1 tablespoon crumbled dried lemon balm
½ teaspoon dried yarrow
1 cup boiling water
stevia (optional)

1. Put the lemon balm and yarrow in a tea ball or infuser. Place in a mug of boiling water.
2. Steep the herbs for 15 minutes.
3. Sweeten with stevia, if desired.
4. Drink this tea 2 to 3 times daily, about 30 minutes before mealtimes.

Chamomile-Clove Tea

YIELD: 1 CUP
STORAGE: NOT RECOMMENDED
TIME: 15 MINUTES

Spicy and naturally sweet, cloves help to short-circuit the brain's desire for excessive amounts of food. Chamomile alleviates associated stress. If bingeing is a problem for you, give this tea a try.

1 teaspoon dried chamomile flowers
5 whole cloves
1¼ cups water
stevia (optional)

1. In a small saucepan, add the chamomile and cloves to the water. Bring to a boil.
2. Reduce the heat to medium-low and simmer the herbs for 10 minutes.
3. Strain into a mug, using the back of a spoon to press excess liquid from the herbs before discarding them.
4. Sweeten with stevia, if desired.
5. Drink hot or iced as often as you like.

INSOMNIA

Insomnia touches every part of your life, making it difficult to function during the day and leading to feelings of hopelessness. Instead of relying on pharmaceuticals to give you the quantity or quality of sleep you need, consider these herbal remedies instead. With no harmful side effects or morning grogginess, they ease you off to slumber gently, keep you asleep, and leave you feeling refreshed when you wake.

Valerian-Hops Tea with Passionflower

YIELD: 1 CUP
STORAGE: NOT RECOMMENDED
TIME: 15 MINUTES

Valerian, hops, and passionflower combine to promote calm, bring deep, restful sleep, and minimize tossing and turning.

1 teaspoon crushed dried hops
1 teaspoon dried passionflower
1 teaspoon dried valerian
1¼ cups water
Honey or stevia (optional)

1. In a small saucepan, add the hops, passionflower, and valerian to the water. Bring to a boil.
2. Reduce the heat to medium-low and simmer the herbs for 10 minutes.
3. Strain into a mug, using the back of a spoon to press the liquid from the herbs before discarding them.
4. Sweeten with honey or stevia, if desired.
5. Drink this tea about 15 minutes before bedtime as often as needed.

❣ Help your mind relax by turning off electronics about 30 minutes beforehand.

Soothing Chamomile-Lavender Bath Salt

YIELD: 1 TREATMENT
STORAGE: NOT RECOMMENDED
TIME: 30 MINUTES

Wash off the stress of the day, relax your body, and prepare your mind for sleep with this fragrant spa treatment. Bathe 1 to 2 hours before bed for best results.

1 cup Epsom salt
5 drops lavender essential oil
3 drops chamomile essential oil

1. Draw a warm bath.
2. Add the Epsom salt and let it dissolve.
3. Add the lavender and chamomile essential oils.
4. Spend 15 to 30 minutes soaking in the tub.

Herbal Bedtime Tea Blend

YIELD: ABOUT 4 CUPS DRIED HERBAL BLEND
STORAGE: AIRTIGHT CONTAINER
TIME: 15 MINUTES

A potent blend that balances the body while inducing restful sleep, this relaxing bedtime tea has a pleasant flavor that most people enjoy.

1½ cups dried chamomile flowers
1 cup crushed dried lemon balm
½ cup crushed dried catnip
½ cup dried oat straw
½ cup dried passionflowers
¼ cup crushed dried hops
1 cup boiling water
Honey or stevia (optional)

1. In an airtight container, combine all the herbs.
2. To brew the tea, use 1 tablespoon of the herbal blend per cup, and place in a tea ball or infuser.
3. In a mug, pour boiling water over the herbs and steep for 15 minutes.
4. Sweeten with honey or stevia, if desired.
5. Drink 1 cup of this tea each night before bed. Store in a cool, dry place.

MEMORY PROBLEMS

Most people think forgetfulness is a sign of brain function, but it's often a result of lifestyle. Forgetfulness could be caused by too little sleep, stress, or even diet. Whatever your reason, natural remedies can often help. While working to alleviate your symptoms, consider the cause of your memory problem. Because forgetfulness can be a sign of a more serious issue, talk to your doctor if it continues or worsens despite your efforts.

Rosemary Smelling Salt

YIELD: 1 OUNCE
STORAGE: SMALL GLASS JAR
TIME: 2 MINUTES

Rosemary essential oil helps to improve memory, reduce anxiety, and promote a sense of overall well-being. Use this treatment alone or in combination with others.

1 ounce coarse sea salt
20 drops rosemary essential oil

1. In a small glass jar, combine the sea salt and the rosemary essential oil.
2. Shake well to blend.
3. Breathe deeply for 20 seconds.
4. Use this remedy regularly, particularly when undertaking cognitive tasks. If you like, you can leave the jar open near your work area. Refresh the smelling salt with more essential oil when the fragrance begins to fade.

Green Tea with Ginseng and Sage

YIELD: 1 CUP
STORAGE: NOT RECOMMENDED
TIME: 15 MINUTES

Green tea, ginseng, and sage combine to boost the chemicals responsible for transmitting messages within your brain.

1 tablespoon crushed dried sage
1 teaspoon chopped dried ginseng root
1 cup boiling water
1 green tea bag
Honey or stevia (optional)
Lemon juice (optional)

1. Place the dried sage and ginseng in a tea ball or infuser. In a mug filled with boiling water add the tea ball and the green tea bag.
2. Steep for 15 minutes.
3. Sweeten with honey or stevia, if desired. Add lemon if the sage flavor seems too strong.
4. Enjoy 2 to 3 cups of this tea each day during the morning and early afternoon hours.

Blueberry-Ginkgo Iced Tea

YIELD: ½ GALLON
STORAGE: REFRIGERATE IN PITCHER
TIME: 15 MINUTES

Blueberries enhance cognitive functioning and boost memory, as does ginkgo biloba. You can find unsweetened blueberry juice at health food stores and some supermarkets, and ginkgo biloba liquid extract is available at health food stores or online.

4 cups boiling water
4 green tea bags
4 cups unsweetened blueberry juice
1¼ tablespoons ginkgo biloba liquid extract
stevia (optional)

1. In a pitcher, combine the water and green tea bags.
2. Steep the tea for 15 minutes. Remove the tea bags.
3. Add the blueberry juice and ginkgo biloba extract.
4. Drink 2 to 3 cups of this tea each day, adding a little stevia to sweeten, if desired.

MOODINESS

Sometimes moodiness is an indicator of mild depression or anxiety, and other times lifestyle issues like stress or diet are to blame. Despite the reason, one thing is for sure: Erratic moods don't feel good to you or the people who interact with you. Work to find out what's behind your feelings while using herbal remedies to treat the symptoms that get in the way of happiness. Getting plenty of sleep can help, as can following a clean, natural diet.

St. John's Wort–Peppermint Tea Blend

YIELD: 4 CUPS DRIED HERBAL TEA BLEND
STORAGE: AIRTIGHT CONTAINER
TIME: 15 MINUTES

St. John's wort and peppermint combine to boost mood over time. You should start to notice positive effects after 3 to 5 weeks of consistent use.

3 cups dried St. John's wort
1 cup crumbled dried peppermint
1 cup boiling water
Honey or stevia (optional)

1. In an airtight container, combine the herbs.
2. To brew, place 1 teaspoon of the herbal blend in a tea ball or infuser, and add to a mug of boiling water.
3. Steep for 15 minutes before drinking.
4. Sweeten with honey or stevia, if desired.
5. Drink 2 cups of this tea daily over an extended period of time.

Passionflower Tonic

YIELD: 1 CUP
STORAGE: NOT RECOMMENDED
TIME: 15 MINUTES

Passionflower relieves tension, nervousness, anxiety, and insomnia. This relaxing tonic boosts mood and is a good one for overall mental health.

1 tablespoon dried passionflower
1 cup water
1 teaspoon honey
1 lemon wedge

1. In a small saucepan, add the passionflower to the water. Bring to a boil and remove from the heat.
2. Steep for 15 minutes. Strain into a mug.
3. Stir in the honey and squeeze the lemon juice into the mug. Drink.
4. Enjoy a cup of this tonic at least once daily to improve your mood.

Lemon-Mandarin Shower Steam

YIELD: 1 TREATMENT
STORAGE: NOT RECOMMENDED
TIME: 15 MINUTES

Lemon, mandarin, and rosemary essential oils combine to enhance your mood. This pleasant treatment is almost certain to give you a more positive outlook on life.

4 drops lemon essential oil
4 drops mandarin essential oil
2 drops rosemary essential oil

1. Drip the lemon, mandarin, and rosemary essential oils onto a washcloth.
2. Place the washcloth on the shower floor, away from the drain.
3. Take your shower as usual, inhaling the aroma while breathing deep.

❦ Enjoy this treatment anytime you feel the need to clear your mind. Follow up with a cup of passionflower tea for even better results.

NERVOUS TENSION

You're living in a modern world; you've likely experienced nervous tension at some time. Whether brought on by financial stress, difficulties in your relationship, or a tough situation at work, this type of tension evaporates quickly when you make relaxation a priority. Instead of unwinding with a cocktail, try these healthy herbal remedies. If you find yourself feeling the effects of nervous tension often, consider talking with your doctor to rule out a more serious problem.

Lemon Balm Tea

YIELD: 1 CUP
STORAGE: NOT RECOMMENDED
TIME: 15 MINUTES

Lemon balm has a fresh, pleasant taste. This tea alleviates tension while leaving you feeling calm and alert.

1 tablespoon dried lemon balm
1 cup boiling water

1. Place the lemon balm in a tea ball or infuser. Add to a mug of boiling water.
2. Steep for 15 minutes.
3. Drink a cup anytime you need to relax but can't take time out for a nap.

Passionflower-Rooibos Iced Tea

YIELD: ½ GALLON
STORAGE: REFRIGERATE IN PITCHER
TIME: 10 MINUTES

Passionflower and rooibos combine to alleviate nervous tension and bring your mood back into balance. Rooibos tea bags are easy to find at health food stores and most supermarkets.

2 tablespoons dried passionflower
4 rooibos tea bags, any flavor
8 cups water

1. In a saucepan, add the passionflower and rooibos tea bags to the water. Bring to a boil.
2. Reduce the heat to medium-low and simmer the herbs for 10 minutes.
3. Remove from the heat, cool, then strain the tea into a pitcher and chill.
4. Sweeten this tea if you like, or flavor it with lemon or vanilla. Drink as much as you like to maintain a state of alert relaxation.

Lavender-Lemon Balm Bath Salt

YIELD: 4 CUPS
STORAGE: AIRTIGHT CONTAINER
TIME: 30 MINUTES

Lavender and lemon balm combine to ease tension. Make this relaxing bath salt ahead of time so you'll have it on hand when needed.

4 cups Epsom salt
½ teaspoon lavender essential oil
½ teaspoon lemon balm essential oil

1. In an airtight container, add the Epsom salt and the lavender and lemon balm essential oils, and use a whisk or fork to blend.
2. Draw a warm bath.
3. Add ¼ cup of the bath salt. Swish until it dissolves.
4. Relax in the bath for 30 minutes.
5. Enjoy this bath salt anytime you feel the need to relax. Store in a dark, cool place between uses.

STRESS

Life is full of frustrations, deadlines, hassles, and demands that all add up to stress, a normal response to events that upset your sense of balance. Sometimes feeling a little pressure works for you by spiking your energy and creating focus so you can get things done. At other times, tension gets out of control, causing problems at work, harming your health, and interfering with relationships. Next time you feel overloaded, try one or two of these remedies.

Chamomile-Tarragon Infusion

YIELD: 1 CUP
STORAGE: NOT RECOMMENDED
TIME: 15 MINUTES

Chamomile and tarragon come together with rosemary and sage to relieve stress, even if only temporarily. This savory infusion pairs well with a variety of foods.

1 teaspoon dried chamomile flowers
1 teaspoon crumbled dried tarragon
½ teaspoon crumbled dried rosemary
½ teaspoon crumbled dried sage
1¼ cups water
Lemon juice (optional)
Honey (optional)

1. In a small saucepan, combine all the ingredients and bring to a boil.
2. Reduce the heat to medium-low and simmer the herbs for 10 minutes.
3. Strain into a mug, using the back of a spoon to press the liquid from the herbs before discarding them.
4. Drink 1 or 2 cups of this infusion anytime you feel stressed. Add some lemon and honey if you prefer a sweet flavor.

Lemon Balm-Orange Iced Tea

YIELD: ½ GALLON
STORAGE: REFRIGERATE IN A PITCHER
TIME: 30 MINUTES

Lemon balm has a faint minty flavor. Not only does it make a wonderfully refreshing iced tea, it helps to alleviate stress and reduce anxiety.

4 tablespoons fresh lemon balm
8 cups water
2 oranges, sliced thinly

1. In a large saucepan, add the lemon balm and water. Bring to a boil.
2. Reduce the heat to medium-low and simmer for 10 minutes.
3. Remove from the heat and cool.
4. Strain into a pitcher, using the back of a spoon to press the liquid from the herbs before discarding them.
5. Add the orange slices and refrigerate until cold.
6. Serve over ice.
7. Drink as much as you want, any time of day.

Frankincense-Lavender Stress Balm

YIELD: 4 OUNCES
STORAGE: GLASS JAR OR TIN
TIME: 15 MINUTES

Rub your temples and pulse points with this fragrant balm next time you're feeling stressed. The combination of frankincense and lavender smells amazing, and it helps you feel less tense.

3 ounces organic olive oil
1 ounce beeswax, grated
20 drops frankincense essential oil
20 drops lavender essential oil

1. In a double boiler over low heat, combine the olive oil and beeswax. Stir gently until the beeswax has melted completely.
2. Remove from the heat and cool for 2 minutes.
3. Add the frankincense and lavender essential oils.
4. Pour into a jar or tin.
5. Cool the balm completely before capping tightly.
6. Apply a thin layer to your temples when feeling stressed. You can also dab this balm onto your pulse points. Store in a cool, dark place.

♥ This is a fantastic remedy for stress-induced headaches. Combine it with other stress-relief techniques for maximum relief.

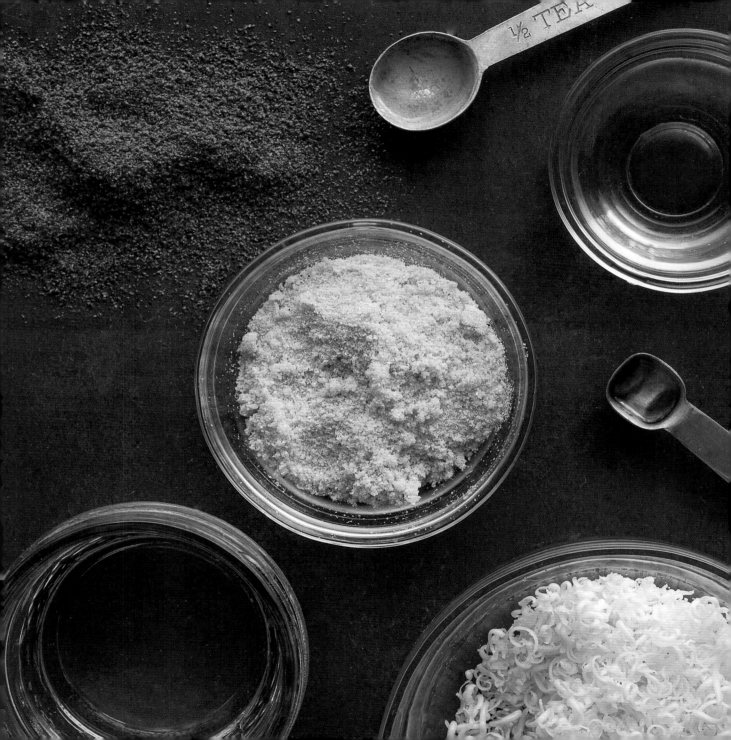

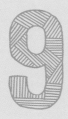

COMMON AILMENTS

ALLERGIES

Sneezing, stuffy sinuses, watery eyes, and other allergy symptoms are part of your body's unique immune response to substances that are not normally harmful. These remedies can be used alone or alongside other alternative or conventional treatments. Start using them as soon as you notice discomfort, and take preventative measures to limit your exposure to allergens. Closing windows and using air purifiers are two helpful steps to take.

Passionflower–Peppermint Infusion

YIELD: 1 CUP
STORAGE: NOT RECOMMENDED
TIME: 15 MINUTES

Passionflower and peppermint combine to open airways and promote relaxation. This infusion has a pleasant taste when served hot or cold.

1 teaspoon dried passionflower
1 teaspoon crushed dried peppermint
1¼ cups water

1. In a small saucepan, add the passionflower and peppermint to the water and bring to a boil.
2. Reduce the heat to medium-low and simmer the herbs for 10 minutes.
3. Strain into a mug, using the back of a spoon to press the liquid from the herbs before discarding them.
4. Drink as soon as you feel allergy symptoms coming on. It is safe to drink as frequently as needed.

Peppermint-Eucalyptus Soak

YIELD: 1 TREATMENT
STORAGE: NOT RECOMMENDED
TIME: 30 MINUTES

Peppermint and eucalyptus combine to bring relief. If seasonal allergies are causing watery eyes, soak two peppermint tea bags in water and place one on each eye while bathing.

7 drops peppermint essential oil
5 drops eucalyptus essential oil

1. Draw a warm bath.
2. Add the peppermint and eucalyptus essential oils.
3. Spend 30 minutes breathing deeply while relaxing in the tub.
4. Enjoy this remedy as often as needed.

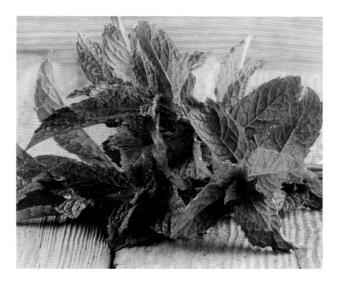

BACKACHE

A comfortable mattress, plenty of exercise, and the right kind of office chair can go a long way toward preventing backaches. In the event of the occasional backache, you'll find that these simple herbal remedies bring comfort. If your back pain was caused by an injury, is chronic, or is severe, see your doctor.

Black Cohosh–Valerian Infusion

YIELD: 1 CUP
STORAGE: NOT RECOMMENDED
TIME: 10 MINUTES

Nothing brings on relaxation and tension relief in muscles quite like the blend of black cohosh and valerian. Take a warm bath or shower to enhance relaxation.

1 tablespoon chopped dried black cohosh root
1 teaspoon dried valerian
1¼ cups water

1. In a small saucepan, add the black cohosh and valerian to the water. Bring to a boil.
2. Reduce the heat to medium-low and simmer the herbs for 10 minutes.
3. Remove from the heat.
4. Strain into a mug, using the back of a spoon to press the liquid from the herbs before discarding them.
5. Drink when you feel a tension backache coming on.

♥ This treatment is likely to make you feel sleepy. Do not use it before driving or doing other tasks that require high levels of concentration.

Ginger-Cayenne Back Balm with Peppermint and Eucalyptus

YIELD: 8 OUNCES
STORAGE: GLASS JAR OR TIN
TIME: 48 HOURS FOR BREWING

Ginger and cayenne bring the heat as peppermint and eucalyptus deliver a relaxing, cooling, refreshing effect deep into sore back muscles. Do not allow this remedy to come into contact with your eyes.

7 ounces organic olive oil
¼ cup cayenne pepper
¼ cup ground ginger
1 ounce grated beeswax
20 drops peppermint essential oil
10 drops eucalyptus essential oil

1. In a jar, add the olive oil, cayenne pepper, and ginger.
2. Cap tightly and put in a warm place for 48 hours. Invert the jar every 8 hours or so to mix the contents together.
3. When the mixture is finished brewing, strain the olive oil into a double boiler. Use the back of a spoon to press the oil from the ground spices before discarding them.
4. Add the beeswax to the double boiler and stir over low heat. Remove from the heat as soon as the beeswax is completely melted. ▶
5. Cool for 2 minutes.
6. Add the peppermint and eucalyptus essential oils, and pour the balm into a jar or tin.
7. Cool completely before capping tightly.
8. Apply a thin layer to painful back muscles and massage well as often as needed. Store in a cool, dry place between uses.

BLISTER

Friction—like the kind caused by those cute new shoes you just had to have—can lead to blisters. Although they look bad and feel worse, it's rarely a good idea to pop these sores as the liquid inside helps protect skin underneath. These herbal remedies can ease the pain when delicate tissue has been pinched or irritated. Watch for signs of infection as your blister heals. Pus or red streaks radiating from the area are signs that you should see your doctor.

Chamomile Blister Balm

YIELD: 4 OUNCES
STORAGE: GLASS JAR OR TIN
TIME: 15 MINUTES

Chamomile soothes pain while helping blisters to heal. This balm is also useful for minor cuts, scrapes, and burns.

3 ounces organic olive oil
1 ounce coconut oil
20 drops chamomile essential oil

1. In a double boiler, combine the olive oil and coconut oil over low heat.
2. Stir until the coconut oil is completely melted.
3. Remove from the heat and cool for 2 minutes.
4. Stir in the chamomile essential oil.
5. Pour into a small jar or tin.
6. Cool completely, then cap tightly.
7. Apply a thin layer of balm to the blister. Top with a bandage or blister pad if needed.
8. Reapply as needed. Keep the balm in a cool, dry place between uses.

Calendula-Lavender Blister Salve

YIELD: 4 OUNCES
STORAGE: GLASS JAR OR TIN
TIME: 15 MINUTES

Use this simple salve for blisters and other minor injuries to skin. It is useful for bug bites, bruises, and burns.

3 ounces coconut oil
1 ounce calendula oil
20 drops lavender essential oil

1. In a double boiler, combine the coconut oil and calendula oil over low heat.
2. Stir until the coconut oil is completely melted.
3. Remove from the heat and cool for 2 minutes.
4. Stir in the lavender essential oil.
5. Pour into a small jar or tin.
6. Cool completely, then cap tightly.
7. Apply a thin layer of salve to the blister. Top with a bandage or blister pad if needed.
8. Reapply as needed. Keep the salve in a cool, dry place between uses.

Cool Tea Tree Compress

YIELD: 1 TREATMENT
STORAGE: NOT RECOMMENDED
TIME: 5 MINUTES

The tea tree essential oil in this simple compress has antibacterial properties to help prevent infection and, because it is an astringent, it will help dry the blister, bringing relief faster.

½ cup crushed ice
½ cup cold water
3 drops tea tree essential oil
1 ice cube

1. In a small dish, combine the crushed ice and cold water.
2. Soak a cotton pad or soft cloth in the ice and water mixture. Wring out the excess moisture.
3. Drip the tea tree essential oil onto the pad or cloth.
4. Apply the pad or cloth to the blister and top it with an ice cube.
5. Use another cloth to hold the ice cube in place for up to 5 minutes.
6. Repeat this treatment 1 to 2 times each day while waiting for a blister to heal. Follow up with a blister balm or salve.

BRUISE

Crashing your bike, taking a spill on the street, or tripping into office furniture leaves you with more than a crushing blow to the ego. It can rupture blood vessels and damage underlying tissues, causing pain, swelling, and a colorful, hard-to-miss mark on the skin. These simple remedies bring relief while helping the injury to heal. If a severe bruise worsens, stays swollen, and continues to be painful despite first aid treatment, see your doctor to rule out an underlying bone injury.

Arnica Salve

YIELD: 8 OUNCES
STORAGE: GLASS JAR OR TIN
TIME: 5 MINUTES

Arnica eases pain and swelling, making it one of the best herbal remedies available for bruises. Make this balm ahead of time and keep it in your first aid kit.

7 ounces organic olive oil
1 ounce beeswax, grated
20 drops arnica essential oil

1. In a double boiler over low heat, combine the olive oil and beeswax. Stir until the beeswax is completely melted.
2. Remove from the heat and cool for 2 minutes.
3. Add the arnica essential oil.
4. Pour into a glass jar or tin and cool completely before capping tightly.
5. Using your fingertips, apply a thin layer of salve to the bruised area.
6. Reapply the salve up to 3 times daily.
7. Use each day until the bruise has faded. Store in a cool, dark place.

St. John's Wort–Calendula Spray

YIELD: 4 OUNCES
STORAGE: GLASS BOTTLE WITH A SPRAY TOP
TIME: 5 MINUTES

St. John's wort essential oil and calendula oil combine with witch hazel to stop pain and swelling while promoting healing.

3½ ounces alcohol-free witch hazel extract
½ ounce calendula oil
20 drops St. John's wort essential oil

1. In a glass bottle, add the witch hazel extract, caledula oil, and St. John's wort essential oil.
2. Cap tightly with a spray top.
3. Shake well before each use.
4. Spray on the bruised area and let it penetrate.
5. Use up to 3 times daily. Keep in a cool, dry place between uses.

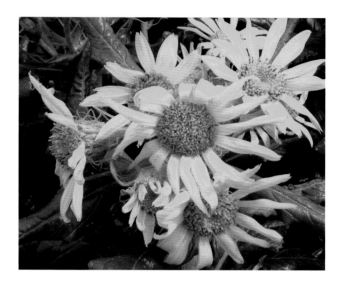

BUG BITES

Warm weather brings opportunities for outdoor fun—and drop-ins by unwanted guests: namely, gnats, mosquitos, and other bugs whose bites can leave pain, itching, and swelling behind. In most cases, herbal remedies zap the irritating sting quickly with no lasting harm done. If, however, you suspect that you have been bitten by a tick or notice symptoms of tick-borne illness, seek medical treatment immediately.

Aloe Vera–Peppermint Gel

YIELD: 8 OUNCES
STORAGE: PLASTIC SQUEEZE BOTTLE
TIME: 5 MINUTES

Aloe vera and peppermint combine to take the sting out of bug bites while relieving swelling. Make a batch ahead of time and keep it in the refrigerator indefinitely.

1 (8-ounce) bottle alcohol-free aloe vera gel
20 drops peppermint essential oil

1. In a large bowl, add the aloe vera gel and peppermint essential oil, and whisk until well blended.
2. Using a funnel, transfer the gel to a plastic squeeze bottle.
3. With your fingertips, apply a small amount to the affected area.
4. Reapply as needed to keep itching and swelling under control.

Lavender-Tea Tree Spray

YIELD: 4 OUNCES
STORAGE: GLASS BOTTLE WITH SPRAY TOP
TIME: 5 MINUTES

With cool witch hazel extract plus anti-inflammatory lavender essential oil and disinfecting tea tree essential oil, this spray soothes insect bites quickly.

4 ounces alcohol-free witch hazel extract
10 drops lavender essential oil
10 drops tea tree essential oil

1. In a glass bottle, combine the witch hazel extract and lavender and tea tree essential oils.
2. Cap tightly with a spray top.
3. Shake well before each use.
4. Spray enough liquid onto the affected area to cover the bug bites.
5. Repeat as necessary to keep discomfort to a minimum. Store in the refrigerator or keep in a cool, dark place between uses.

Soothing Aloe and Calendula Salve

YIELD: ABOUT 1 OUNCE
STORAGE: REFRIGERATE IN SEALED CONTAINER
TIME: 15 MINUTES

Calendula helps stop the itching associated with bug bites by easing inflammation. Aloe and lavender help to heal damaged skin and prevent infection. Before going camping, whip up a batch and keep it in the refrigerator or in a cooler—odds are, you'll need it!

½ tablespoon calendula oil
½ tablespoon coconut oil, melted
1 tablespoons alcohol-free aloe vera gel
10 drops lavender essential oil

1. In a small dish, combine the calendula oil and coconut oil.
2. Add the aloe vera gel and the lavender essential oil.
3. Use a small whisk or fork to stir every few minutes until the oils and aloe gel stop separating from one another.
4. Cap tightly and store in the refrigerator.
5. To use, apply a dab onto each bug bite with your fingertip.
6. Use as often as needed. Top with a cold compress to help stop any swelling.

BURN

Even a seemingly minor incident, like a kitchen accident or a slip of the curling iron, can cause a painful burn. In most cases, small injuries can be easily treated at home. The first step in treating a burn is to cool it off by immersing the injured area in cold water for a few minutes. Afterward, use one of these quick herbal remedies to ease the pain and help your skin heal faster.

Burn-No-More Oil

YIELD: 1 TREATMENT
STORAGE: GLASS ESSENTIAL OIL BOTTLE
TIME: 1 MINUTE

For minor burns, straight lavender essential oil is one of the best natural remedies available. Used immediately, it eases pain and helps to prevent scarring.

2 drops lavender essential oil

1. Drip the essential oil directly from the bottle onto your burn.
2. Leave the essential oil in place.
3. Repeat 2 to 3 times daily while your burn is healing.

Fresh Aloe Vera Leaf

YIELD: 1 TREATMENT
STORAGE: NOT RECOMMENDED
TIME: 20 MINUTES

Fresh aloe vera gel cools burns quickly while helping skin heal. Aloe vera is easy to grow indoors. Keeping one of these plants ensures you'll always have a quick remedy on hand.

1 aloe vera leaf

1. Using a sharp knife, split the aloe vera leaf open lengthwise.
2. Place the leaf over your burn, gel side down.
3. With a soft cloth, gently bind the leaf to your burn.
4. Leave the leaf in place for 20 minutes.
5. Using cool water, gently rinse away any excess aloe vera gel.
6. Repeat the treatment 2 to 3 times daily while your burn is healing.

Cool Chamomile-Aloe Compress

YIELD: 1 TREATMENT
STORAGE: NOT RECOMMENDED
TIME: 15 MINUTES

Chamomile essential oil, aloe, and cold water help keep fresh burns from blistering. If you're in doubt about the seriousness of a burn, seek emergency medical treatment after cooling the burned area.

½ teaspoon aloe vera gel
2 drops chamomile essential oil
1 cup cold water
2 drops lavender essential oil (optional)

1. Run cold tap water over the burn for 5 minutes.
2. In a small dish, combine the aloe vera gel and chamomile essential oil.
3. With a fingertip, apply the aloe and chamomile to the burn.
4. Wet a soft cloth in the water, wring it out, and place it over the burned area. Leave in place for at least 5 to 10 minutes.
5. Allow the burned area to air dry after the compress is removed.
6. For best results, follow up by placing 1 or 2 drops of lavender essential oil onto the affected area after it is dry. Repeat as often as needed.

CANKER SORE/ COLD SORE

Cold sores and canker sores have some things in common, but it's important to keep in mind that cold sores are caused by the herpes virus while canker sores are usually caused by friction or irritation. If you feel an itching or tingling sensation before a sore develops, it is likely that you are dealing with a cold sore rather than a canker sore. These natural treatments can be used alone or alongside over-the-counter remedies.

Lemon Balm-Licorice Infusion

YIELD: 1 CUP
STORAGE: NOT RECOMMENDED
TIME: 10 MINUTES

Lemon balm and licorice are effective agents against the virus that causes cold sores. If fresh lemon balm is not available, use freeze-dried lemon balm instead.

1 tablespoon chopped fresh lemon balm
1 teaspoon chopped dried licorice root
1¼ cups water

1. In a small saucepan, add the lemon balm and the licorice to the water. Bring to a boil.
2. Reduce the heat to medium-low and simmer the herbs for 10 minutes.
3. Strain into a mug, using the back of a spoon to press the liquid from the herbs before discarding them.
4. Drink hot or iced.
5. Enjoy this infusion 3 to 4 times daily as soon as you notice the tingling that precedes a cold sore.

Licorice Mouth Rinse

YIELD: 1 CUP
STORAGE: GLASS BOTTLE
TIME: 10 MINUTES

Licorice root helps canker sores heal faster. If you are using another remedy alongside this one, apply it after rinsing.

1 cup warm water
½ teaspoon powdered licorice root

1. In a measuring cup, add the warm water and powdered licorice root, and whisk to blend thoroughly.
2. With a funnel, transfer the mouth rinse to a glass bottle.
3. Use 1 tablespoon per treatment. Hold the solution in your mouth and swish gently for 2 to 3 minutes before spitting out.
4. Repeat each morning and evening until your canker sore has healed.

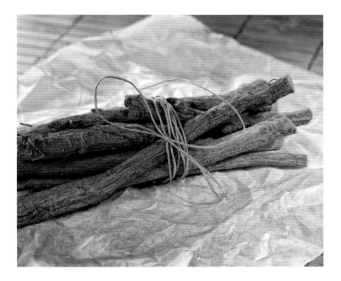

COLD & FLU

Caused by viruses and spread by contact with everyday objects, the common cold and seasonal flu can be difficult to prevent and even harder to get rid of. While there is no cure for these illnesses, you can use a variety of herbal remedies to ease your symptoms and perhaps shorten the duration. If symptoms are severe, see your doctor for something stronger.

Comforting Peppermint-Echinacea Tea

YIELD: 1 CUP
STORAGE: NOT RECOMMENDED
TIME: 15 MINUTES

This soothing tea is chock full of immunity boosters to stave off all-too-familiar cold and flu symptoms and kick the viruses to the curb. Start using it as soon as you notice symptoms.

1 teaspoon dried peppermint leaves
1 tablespoon dried echinacea root
1 cup boiling water
Honey or stevia (optional)

1. Put the peppermint leaves and echinacea root in a tea ball or infuser. Place the herbs in a mug of boiling water.
2. Steep for 10 to 15 minutes.
3. Sweeten with a little honey or stevia, if desired.
4. Repeat 3 times daily while experiencing cold or flu symptoms.

Eucalyptus-Sage Bath Salt

YIELD: 1 CUP
STORAGE: GLASS JAR
TIME: 20 MINUTES

Proven cold fighters eucalyptus and sage tag team to open blocked nasal passages and ease chest congestion. Meanwhile, a warm bath will help you to relax while alleviating body aches.

1 cup Epsom salt
20 drops eucalyptus essential oil
10 drops sage essential oil

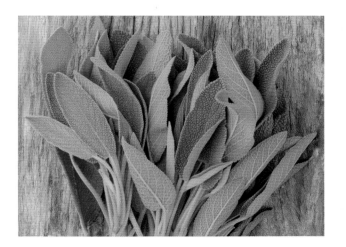

1. In a medium bowl, add the Epsom salt and the eucalyptus and sage essential oils. With a spoon, stir well to combine.
2. Using a funnel, transfer the bath salt to a glass jar with a tight-fitting lid.
3. To use, run a warm bath and dissolve ¼ cup of the bath salt in the tub.
4. Soak for 20 minutes daily while recuperating from a cold or the flu.

CONSTIPATION

If you've ever devoured an entire cheese plate, you know that no matter how healthy you are, nearly everyone gets constipated at some time. Uncomfortable and frustrating, constipation occurs when waste becomes difficult to pass. If you strain during bowel movements, have hard stools, or have two or fewer bowel movements over the course of a week, give these treatments a try. Increasing water intake, eating more fiber, and exercising can help, too.

Ginger-Fennel Infusion

YIELD: 1 CUP
STORAGE: NOT RECOMMENDED
TIME: 20 MINUTES

Ginger and fennel increase blood flow to the intestinal tract and gently alleviate constipation. This remedy may ease other gastrointestinal symptoms, too, like gas, cramps, or bloating.

2 tablespoons peeled, grated fresh ginger
1 tablespoon fennel seeds
1 tablespoon honey
1¼ cups water

1. In a small saucepan, add the ginger, fennel, and honey to the water. Bring to a boil.
2. Reduce the heat to medium-low and simmer the spices for 15 minutes.
3. Strain into a mug, using the back of a spoon to press the liquid from the spices before discarding them.
4. Drink 2 to 3 cups daily while constipated.

♥ This infusion has a spicy flavor that some find overpowering. If it seems too strong, mix it with a cup of water or apple juice before drinking the entire dose.

Chamomile-Rose Hip Infusion

YIELD: 1 CUP
STORAGE: NOT RECOMMENDED
TIME: 15 MINUTES

This stimulating trio of chamomile, rose hips, and slippery elm works while you sleep, activating the digestive tract and bringing relief from constipation as you get your Zzzs.

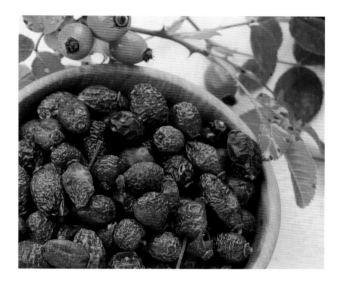

1 tablespoon dried chamomile flowers
1 tablespoon chopped dried rose hips
2 teaspoons slippery elm powder
1¼ cups water

1. In a small saucepan, add the chamomile, rose hips, and slippery elm powder to the water. Bring to a boil.
2. Reduce the heat to medium-low and simmer the herbs for 10 minutes.
3. Strain into a mug, using the back of a spoon to press the liquid from the herbs before discarding them.
4. Drink this infusion before bed.

🌱 In severe cases of constipation, drink up to 4 cups of the infusion beginning late in the afternoon. You should have relief by morning.

CUTS & SCRAPES

These simple remedies are best for small injuries, the kinds of cuts and scrapes you get by going about your normal day in the kitchen, during the commute, or working at the office (paper cuts, this means you). Start by cleaning the affected area, and then apply the salve or poultice. If a wound is deep, involves severe bleeding, or contains deeply embedded dirt, gravel, or splinters, you may need professional treatment.

Lavender–Eucalyptus Salve

YIELD: 8 OUNCES
STORAGE: GLASS JAR OR TIN
TIME: 15 MINUTES

Lavender and eucalyptus combine with calendula to prevent infection while helping minor cuts and scrapes to heal faster.

- **3 ounces coconut oil**
- **1 ounce beeswax, grated**
- **3 ounces calendula oil**
- **30 drops lavender essential oil**
- **20 drops eucalyptus essential oil**

1. In a double boiler, combine the coconut oil and beeswax. Stir gently until the beeswax is completely melted.
2. Remove from the heat.
3. Add the calendula oil.
4. Cool for 2 minutes.
5. Add the lavender and eucalyptus essential oils.
6. Pour into a glass jar or tin and cool completely before capping tightly.
7. Use your fingertips to apply a thin layer of salve to the affected area.
8. Repeat 2 to 3 times daily until wounds heal. Store in a cool, dark place between uses.

Burdock-Yarrow Poultice

YIELD: 1 POULTICE
STORAGE: NOT RECOMMENDED
TIME: 30 MINUTES

Burdock and yarrow combine with comfrey to ease pain and promote healing while cleansing wounds.

1 tablespoon chopped dried burdock root
or 3 tablespoons chopped fresh burdock root
1 tablespoon dried yarrow
or 3 tablespoons fresh yarrow
1 tablespoon dried comfrey
or 3 tablespoons fresh comfrey
½ cup water
4 drops lavender essential oil (optional)
4 drops eucalyptus essential oil (optional)

1. In a small saucepan, add the burdock, yarrow, and comfrey to the water. Bring to a boil.
2. Simmer the herbs for 10 minutes.
3. Strain into a shallow bowl, using the back of a spoon to press the liquid from the herbs before discarding them.
4. Add the lavender and eucalyptus essential oils, if using.
5. Dip a soft cloth into the bowl, soak it, and wring out the excess liquid.
6. Place the poultice over the affected area.
7. Leave the treatment in place for 20 minutes, refreshing the poultice with additional liquid as needed.
8. Repeat in 1 hour if needed. Switch to a salve when a scab forms.

Coconut-Lavender First Aid Salve

YIELD: 1 OUNCE
STORAGE: JAR OR TIN IN REFRIGERATOR
OR COOL, DRY PLACE
TIME: 5 MINUTES

Make a batch of this couldn't-be-easier salve to keep on hand for treating minor wounds. Coconut oil contains medium-chain fatty acids (MCFAs) that help cuts and scrapes heal faster, while lavender essential oil is a powerful antibacterial agent.

1 ounce coconut oil, melted
20 drops lavender essential oil

1. In a small container, combine the melted coconut oil and lavender essential oil.
2. Cap tightly and refrigerate or store in a cool, dry place.
3. If needed immediately, clean the wound with soap and water, and rinse it. Then apply a thin layer of the salve with a clean fingertip. Or, if you plan to apply an adhesive bandage, just put a dab on the bandage before using it to cover the wound.
4. Apply the salve to the wound 2 to 3 times daily.

DIARRHEA

You're probably not reading this section for a definition of diarrhea, rather a remedy for the uncomfortable cramps, abdominal bloating, and severe sense of urgency that sends you running for the nearest restroom. Instead of settling for chalky solutions from the drugstore, try these herbal treatments instead. Take care of yourself by staying well hydrated while waiting for your symptoms to improve.

Raspberry Leaf–Prunella Infusion

YIELD: 1 CUP
STORAGE: NOT RECOMMENDED
TIME: 15 MINUTES

Need relief stat? Raspberry leaf, prunella, and slippery elm have got your back. They work fast to stave off cramps, dehydration, and frequent trips to the bathroom. Surprisingly, this treatment also happens to work for sore throats.

1 tablespoon crumbled dried raspberry leaf
1 tablespoon dried prunella
2 teaspoons slippery elm powder
1¼ cups water

1. In a small saucepan, add the raspberry leaf, prunella, and slippery elm powder, and stir to blend. Add the water and bring to a boil.
2. Reduce the heat to medium-low and simmer the herbs for 10 minutes.
3. Strain into a mug, using the back of a spoon to press the liquid from the herbs before discarding them.
4. Drink 1 cup of this infusion every 2 hours. You can drink up to 4 cups daily to stop diarrhea.

Comfrey-Mullein Tea

YIELD: 1 CUP
STORAGE: NOT RECOMMENDED
TIME: 15 MINUTES

This fab four not only stops diarrhea fast, but drinking them as a tea helps prevent dehydration, a frequent side effect. If sipping this tea in the late afternoon or evening, omit the caffeine-rich green tea (unless you want to pull an all-nighter).

- **1 teaspoon dried comfrey**
- **1 teaspoon dried mullein leaf**
- **1 teaspoon crumbled dried peppermint leaves**
- **1¼ cups boiling water**
- **1 green tea bag**
- **Honey or stevia (optional)**

1. Put the comfrey, mullein leaf, and peppermint in a tea ball or infuser. Place in a mug of boiling water with the green tea bag.
2. Steep the herbs for 15 minutes.
3. Add honey or stevia, if desired. Drink up to 4 times daily when recovering from diarrhea.

Carob Smoothie

YIELD: 1 SERVING
STORAGE: NOT RECOMMENDED
TIME: 5 MINUTES

Carob powder, a popular alternative to cocoa powder, is a nutritious herbal food source that has a wonderful chocolate taste. Blended into a smoothie with fiber-rich banana, nourishing yogurt with probiotics, and honey, it can help put an end to diarrhea. If preparing this drink for a child under 12 years of age, cut the amount of carob down to 2 teaspoons and leave the rest of the ingredients the same.

- **¼ cup water**
- **¼ cup plain yogurt with live, active cultures**
- **1½ tablespoons carob powder**
- **1 tablespoon honey**
- **1 ripe banana**

1. In a blender, combine all the ingredients in the order shown.
2. Blend until smooth, adding a little more water to thin, if preferred. Serve immediately.
3. Drink this smoothie twice daily while suffering from diarrhea, preferably once in the morning and once in the afternoon, before dinner.

EARACHE

When fluids build up in the middle ear, the pressure can be a pain in the, well, ear. The issue commonly accompanies a cold or the flu or occurs after swimming. Herbal remedies tend to be the best medicine for minor earaches. If pain increases, a fever develops, or other symptoms rear their heads, be sure to visit your doctor. Antibiotics may be necessary.

Garlic Drops

YIELD: 1 TREATMENT
STORAGE: NOT RECOMMENDED
TIME: 5 MINUTES

Garlic's extraordinary anti-inflammatory and antibiotic properties make it a natural choice for killing bacteria in ears and easing the pressure from built-up fluid. Take these on the go for relief throughout the day.

1 clove garlic, peeled

1. Using a garlic press, hold the garlic clove over a small bowl.
2. Crush the garlic, extracting the juice into the bowl.
3. Use a dropper to pick up the juice.
4. Tilt your head to the side so the painful ear is facing up.
5. Drip the garlic juice into your ear.
6. Place a cotton ball over the ear opening. Leave the cotton ball in place for 5 minutes.
7. Repeat this treatment twice daily for up to 3 days. Discontinue immediately if the pain worsens or does not seem to improve after the first 2 treatments.

Hot Peppermint Compress

YIELD: 1 TREATMENT
STORAGE: NOT RECOMMENDED
TIME: 15 MINUTES

Peppermint essential oil helps alleviate ear pain, as does moist heat. This treatment can be used on its own or alongside antibiotics. Prepare the hot water bottle before you apply the remedy.

3 drops olive oil
3 drops peppermint essential oil

1. Fill a bottle with hot water. Wrap it in a moist towel.
2. In a spoon, combine the olive oil and peppermint essential oil.
3. With your fingertips, apply the oil to the outside of the ear, the area behind the ear, and the soft tissue just behind your jaw. Do not put the oil inside your ear.
4. Relax for 15 minutes while resting the hot water bottle on your ear.
5. Repeat 2 to 3 times daily while recovering from an ear infection.

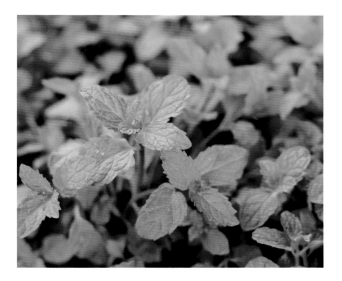

FEVER

Sounds counterintuitive, but running a temperature isn't just a symptom of sickness, it's a natural healing function. By dialing up the heat, the body triggers the immune system to destroy viruses and infectious bacteria. Smart, huh? These treatments allow your fever to run its course while stimulating sweat glands to eliminate toxins and keeping your body temps from getting dangerously high. Seek medical treatment if your fever exceeds 102 degrees Fahrenheit or lasts longer than three days.

Peppermint-Yarrow Tea

YIELD: 4 CUPS
STORAGE: REFRIGERATE IN GLASS CANNING JAR
TIME: 4 HOURS FOR BREWING

Yarrow attacks fever on two fronts: It helps cool the body by making you sweat, and it lowers temps with salicylic acid, an active ingredient in aspirin. Peppermint's cooling effects help clear sinuses.

1 ounce dried peppermint leaves, 3 ounces fresh peppermint leaves, or 1 peppermint tea bag
1 ounce dried yarrow or 3 ounces fresh yarrow
4 cups boiling water

1. Place the peppermint and yarrow in a heat-resistant bowl.
2. Pour the boiling water on top of the herbs.
3. Cover the bowl.
4. Let the infusion sit at room temperature for 4 hours.
5. Strain the liquid into a glass canning jar. Use the back of a spoon to press excess liquid from the herbs before discarding them.
6. Drink 1 cup of the infusion 3 times daily for up to 3 days, storing the jar in the refrigerator between doses.

Cool Peppermint Compress

YIELD: 1 TREATMENT
STORAGE: NOT RECOMMENDED
TIME: 20 MINUTES

Peppermint essential oil has a wonderful cooling effect that relieves the discomfort of a fever. While this treatment won't break you out in a temperature-reducing sweat, it makes a low fever easier to live with.

½ cup cool water
6 drops peppermint essential oil

1. In a large bowl, combine the water with the peppermint essential oil.
2. Soak a facecloth or hand towel in the bowl. Wring out excess moisture.
3. Fold the cloth to fit your forehead.
4. Recline or lie comfortably for 15 minutes, refolding the cloth to permit heat to dissipate as needed.
5. Repeat as often as you like. Try alternating the compress's position from your forehead to the back of your neck for additional relief.

Cooling Triple Oil Bath

YIELD: 1 TREATMENT
STORAGE: NOT RECOMMENDED
TIME: 20 TO 30 MINUTES

Lavender, rosemary, and peppermint essential oils combine with cool water to bring relief from fever while offering comfort by way of their lovely scent. If you're missing one or two of the essential oils, don't worry. Simply relaxing in a lukewarm bath with just one of these oils can help you feel better fast.

1 tablespoon olive, almond, or flaxseed oil
6 drops lavender essential oil
6 drops rosemary essential oil
6 drops peppermint essential oil

1. Draw a bath. The water should feel lukewarm to cool, not cold.
2. Add the oil and essential oils, and submerge your body in it as far as possible.
3. Soak in the tub for 20 to 30 minutes.
4. After toweling off, take a short nap or go directly to bed (if bathing in the evening).
5. Enjoy this bath treatment 1 to 3 times daily while fever persists. If fever does not reduce by the third day, see your doctor.

FLATULENCE

Flatulence may be normal, but that doesn't mean it's a welcomed condition, especially when accompanied by unpleasant symptoms. These treatments bring relief within a few hours for occasional gas and bloating. Seek medical treatment if the problem is constant or accompanied by abdominal pain and swelling, as it may be a sign of an underlying illness.

Ginger-Clove Infusion

YIELD: 1 CUP
STORAGE: NOT RECOMMENDED
TIME: 10 MINUTES

Digestive systems love ginger and clove. Together they reduce gas in the digestive tract and ease flatulence symptoms. Unfortunately this treatment won't work instantly, but it is reliable.

2 tablespoons peeled, grated fresh ginger root
4 whole cloves
1¼ cups water
Honey or stevia (optional)

1. In a small saucepan, add the ginger and cloves to the water. Bring to a boil.
2. Reduce the heat to medium-low and let the spices simmer for 10 minutes.
3. Strain into a mug, using the back of a spoon to press the liquid from the spices before discarding them.
4. Add honey or stevia, if desired, and drink.

♥ This infusion is also a good choice for gastrointestinal issues such as indigestion.

Peppermint Tea

YIELD: 1 CUP
STORAGE: NOT RECOMMENDED
TIME: 15 MINUTES

Sip peppermint tea after your last meal of the day if flatulence tends to be a problem for you. Easy to make with fresh or dried peppermint or a tea bag, it makes a good post-meal remedy for stopping gas before it starts.

**1 tablespoon dried peppermint leaves,
 3 tablespoons fresh peppermint leaves,
 or 1 peppermint teabag
1 cup boiling water
Honey or stevia (optional)**

1. Put the loose peppermint in a tea ball or infuser. Add to a mug of boiling water.
2. Steep the herbs for 15 minutes.
3. Add honey or stevia, if desired.
4. Drink.

❦ Peppermint tea stops flatulence when it is already in progress, and if you drink it after eating food that brings gas with it, it can help stop flatulence from starting.

Peppermint-Clary Sage Abdominal Massage Blend

YIELD: 4 OUNCES
STORAGE: DARK-COLORED GLASS BOTTLE
TIME: 5 MINUTES

Massaging the abdomen soothes nerves, alleviates upset stomach, and improves the digestive process, helping to put a stop to gastric disturbances. This blend is ideal for times when you've overindulged in rich food or had too much to drink.

**4 ounces organic olive oil
28 drops peppermint essential oil
16 drops clary sage essential oil
12 drops caraway essential oil**

1. In a dark-colored glass bottle, combine all of the ingredients. Shake well to blend.
2. Apply 1 teaspoon of the blend to your hands and rub them together.
3. Using firm pressure, massage your abdomen, beginning under the ribcage and working counter-clockwise around the entire abdominal area, rubbing in small circles as you go.
4. Continue the process for up to 5 minutes.
5. You may notice more gas for a few minutes as things work their way out of your system. You should feel more like yourself again within 10 to 15 minutes of ending the massage. Use as often as needed. Store in a cool, dry place.

GASTRO-INTESTINAL DISTRESS (GI DISTRESS)

There are a number of issues from minor to more severe that can lead to gastrointestinal distress: certain foods, unhealthy bacteria, food poisoning, or an infectious disease. Simple herbal remedies work well in many cases. See your doctor if your problems are frequent or severe, as GI symptoms can be indicative of a serious medical problem.

Goldenseal-Comfrey Infusion

YIELD: 1 CUP
STORAGE: NOT RECOMMENDED
TIME: 15 MINUTES

Goldenseal and comfrey promote circulation within the GI tract, relieving distress and improving digestion. They also have a mild antimicrobial effect, helping to bring intestinal flora back into healthy balance.

1 tablespoon dried goldenseal
1 tablespoon dried comfrey
1 tablespoon honey
1¼ cups water

1. In a small saucepan, add the goldenseal, comfrey, and honey to the water. Bring to a boil.
2. Reduce the heat to medium-low and simmer the herbs for 10 minutes.
3. Strain into a mug, using the back of a spoon to press the liquid from the herbs before discarding them.
4. Drink 1 cup 3 times daily while recovering from GI distress.

Licorice-Peppermint Infusion

YIELD: 1 CUP
STORAGE: NOT RECOMMENDED
TIME: 15 MINUTES

Intestinal pain and spasms don't stand a chance against this antioxidant-rich roundup of licorice, peppermint, fennel, and slippery elm. Even better, you'll love the refreshingly sweet flavor courtesy of this unique blend.

1 teaspoon chopped licorice root
1 tablespoon crumbled dried peppermint leaves
½ teaspoon fennel seeds
1 teaspoon slippery elm powder
1¼ cups water

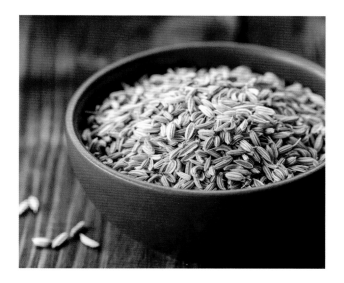

1. In a small saucepan, combine the licorice root, peppermint, fennel seeds, and slippery elm powder, stirring to blend. Add the water and bring to a boil.
2. Reduce the heat to medium-low and simmer the herbs for 10 minutes.
3. Strain into a mug, using the back of a spoon to press the liquid from the herbs before discarding them.
4. Drink as often as you like. Have a cup after dinner to improve digestion.

HEADACHE & MIGRAINE

Stress, tension, exposure to irritants, and lack of sleep are just some of the many reasons headaches and migraines happen. Next time you experience one, try these herbal treatments, either on their own or alongside other therapies. See your doctor if you suffer from these ailments frequently, as an underlying illness could be to blame.

Peppermint Salve

YIELD: 4 OUNCES
STORAGE: GLASS JAR OR TIN
TIME: 15 MINUTES

When applied topically, peppermint helps ease pain by increasing blood flow to the head and neck. This remedy is particularly useful for tension headaches.

3 ounces organic olive oil
1 ounce beeswax, grated
1 teaspoon peppermint essential oil

1. In a double boiler, combine the olive oil and beeswax. Stir gently until the beeswax is completely melted.
2. Remove from the heat and cool for 2 minutes.
3. Add the peppermint essential oil and stir in.
4. Pour into a jar or tin.
5. Cool completely before capping tightly.
6. Apply a thin layer to the back of your neck, your temples, and the area behind your ears.
7. Massage gently for 1 minute while breathing deeply.
8. Reapply every 10 to 15 minutes until the headache subsides. Store in a cool, dark place.

Soothing Valerian Tea with Hops and Peppermint

YIELD: ABOUT 1 CUP
STORAGE: NOT RECOMMENDED
TIME: 15 MINUTES

Valerian, hops, and peppermint join forces to relax the body and mind. If you enjoy this tea, make a larger batch of blended dried herbs and store it in an airtight container for easy prep next time a migraine hits.

1 tablespoon crushed dried hops
1 tablespoon crushed dried peppermint leaves
1 tablespoon dried valerian root
1¼ cups boiling water

1. Put the hops, peppermint leaves, and valerian root in a tea ball or strainer. Place in a mug with the boiling water.
2. Steep the herbs for 15 minutes.
3. Drink the tea while relaxing.

♟ This tea can be sedating. Do not drink it before driving or doing other tasks that require concentration.

Lavender-Peppermint Compress

YIELD: 1 TREATMENT
STORAGE: NOT RECOMMENDED
TIME: 15 MINUTES

Choose a hot compress if you are suffering from a tension headache, and use a cold compress if your headache is accompanied by a fever or nausea. If you are suffering from a migraine, alternating between hot and cold compresses can bring quick relief.

3 drops lavender essential oil
1 drop peppermint essential oil
2 drops valerian essential oil (optional)
Ice pack for cold compress or hot water and facecloth for hot compress

1. In a small dish, combine the essential oils.
2. Using your fingertips, apply the blend to the area where pain is prevalent.
3. Lay a cloth over your head and apply the compress.
4. Keep the treatment in place for 10 to 15 minutes.
5. Repeat once an hour while suffering from a headache or migraine.

HEARTBURN/ INDIGESTION

With major burning, bloating, and other painful symptoms, heartburn and indigestion can cause serious discomfort, disrupting your daily routine or keeping you from getting the sleep you need. These teas are no magic cure for the condition, but they'll provide incredible relief from the symptoms. That said, see your doctor if you suffer from these problems frequently, as a serious underlying medical problem could be to blame.

Chamomile-Sage Tea with Peppermint

YIELD: 1 CUP
STORAGE: NOT RECOMMENDED
TIME: 15 MINUTES

This threesome scores major points for relieving digestive discomfort. Its taste? Not so much. Mask the strong herbal flavor with honey or stevia to sweeten it if needed.

1 tablespoon dried chamomile flowers
1 tablespoon crushed dried sage
1 tablespoon crushed dried peppermint leaves
1¼ cups boiling water
Honey or stevia (optional)

1. Put the chamomile, sage, and peppermint in a tea ball or infuser. Place in a mug with the boiling water.
2. Steep the herbs for 15 minutes.
3. Add honey or stevia, if using.
4. Drink the tea while relaxing.

❦ If you find this tea helpful, make a larger batch and keep the blend in a sealed container.

Ginger Tea

YIELD: 1 CUP
STORAGE: NOT RECOMMENDED
TIME: 15 MINUTES

Faster than popping an over-the-counter pill, this tea quickly alleviates gas in the digestive tract after a meal. Because ginger boasts a delicious spicy-sweet taste, no one will know you're sipping it to prevent an uncomfortable social situation.

1 tablespoon peeled, grated fresh ginger root
1 cup boiling water
Honey or stevia (optional)

1. Place the grated ginger in a tea ball or infuser. Add to a mug of boiling water.
2. Steep the ginger for 15 minutes.
3. Sweeten with honey or stevia, if desired.
4. Drink the tea while relaxing.

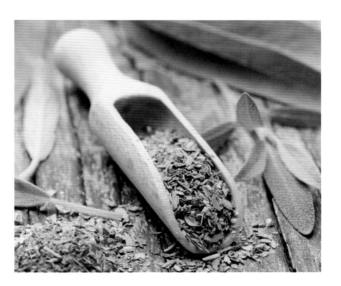

❣ This tea makes a good after-dinner drink. Enjoy it as often as you like.

HEMORRHOIDS

Hemorrhoids form when excess pressure is placed on the veins inside the anal canal or near the opening of the anus. This can happen during pregnancy, or it can happen because of straining due to constipation or diarrhea. Use these herbal remedies to bring relief. See your doctor if symptoms worsen or fail to improve.

Soothing Witch Hazel–Geranium Wipes

YIELD: 30 WIPES
STORAGE: GLASS JAR OR RESEALABLE PLASTIC CONTAINER
TIME: 5 MINUTES

The incredible anti-inflammatory, antibacterial, antifungal, antiseptic, and antihemorrhagic forces in these wipes shrink swollen tissue, banish itching, and temper the burning associated with hemorrhoids.

¼ cup alcohol-free witch hazel extract
10 drops geranium essential oil
30 cotton cosmetic pads

1. In a jar or resealable plastic container, combine the witch hazel extract and geranium essential oil.
2. Swirl the container for 10 seconds to blend.
3. Stack the cotton cosmetic pads in the container.
4. Cover tightly and invert to soak the pads.
5. After bathing or showering, apply a pad to the anus.
6. Press lightly for 5 to 10 seconds to ensure the liquid contacts the irritated area.
7. Repeat as often as needed to obtain relief. Keep in a cool, dark place.

Plantain-Prunella Salve with Lavender

YIELD: ABOUT 8 OUNCES
STORAGE: GLASS JAR OR TIN
TIME: 48 HOURS FOR BREWING

The bad news is that this recipe takes 2 days to formulate, but the upside is that using it brings rapid relief. Make a big batch in advance to streamline healing and keep it on hand for treating minor wounds and burns, too.

7 ounces organic olive oil
4 tablespoons crushed dried plantain leaves
4 tablespoons crushed dried prunella
1 tablespoon grated beeswax
20 drops lavender essential oil

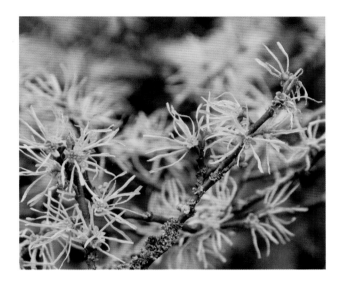

1. In a jar with a tight-fitting lid, combine the olive oil, plantain leaves, and prunella.
2. Cap tightly and put in a warm place for 48 hours.
3. Strain the olive oil into a double boiler, using the back of a spoon to press as much oil as possible from the herbs before discarding them.
4. Add the grated beeswax. Over low heat, stir until the wax melts completely.
5. Remove from the heat and cool for 2 minutes.
6. Add the lavender essential oil.
7. Pour the salve into the jar or tin and cool completely before capping tightly.
8. After bathing or showering, apply a thin layer to the anus.
9. Repeat as often as needed to obtain relief.

HIVES

If you get hives, you know what they look like, but you may not know what's caused them. Could be a number of factors, like vitamin supplements, drugs (aspirin or penicillin), foods (berries, nuts, chocolate), and even heat, cold, or sunlight. Regardless of the cause, the symptoms are the same: swollen areas that usually itch like crazy. Irritation can last anywhere from just a few hours to several days. Try these remedies while working with your doctor to determine which allergen or irritant to avoid in the future.

Cooling Peppermint Bath

YIELD: 1 TREATMENT
STORAGE: NOT RECOMMENDED
TIME: 30 MINUTES

While this treatment is a little bit messy, it works well. Ground oats and peppermint combine to ease the painful itch and swelling associated with hives.

10 drops peppermint essential oil
¼ cup oat flour

1. Draw a warm bath.
2. Add the peppermint essential oil.
3. Sprinkle the oat flour onto the surface of the water.
4. Spend 30 minutes soaking.
5. Repeat twice daily while recovering from hives.

Aloe Vera–Witch Hazel Spray

YIELD: 4 OUNCES
STORAGE: SPRAY BOTTLE
TIME: 5 MINUTES

This fast-working aloe vera and witch hazel twosome teams up in a handy spray to ease the itching, swelling, and redness of hives in hard-to-reach spots like your back. Use this treatment alone or alongside others.

3 ounces alcohol-free witch hazel extract
1 ounce alcohol-free aloe vera gel
10 drops peppermint essential oil

1. In a spray bottle, combine the witch hazel extract, aloe vera gel, and peppermint essential oil.
2. Shake well to blend.
3. Spray liberally on affected area.
4. Repeat as often as needed to keep itching to a minimum. Store in a cool, dark place.

Nettle-Chamomile Wash

YIELD: 1 TREATMENT
STORAGE: NOT RECOMMENDED
TIME: 5 MINUTES

Though this remedy may seem counterintuitive, nettles are among the best herbs for easing the itch and redness associated with hives. Nettle offers both anti-inflammatory and antihistamine action, aiding your body in moderating its response to allergens.

1 cup boiling water
1 tablespoon dried stinging nettle leaves
1 teaspoon olive oil
4 drops chamomile essential oil

1. In a small bowl, combine the boiling water and stinging nettle leaves. Allow it to steep until cool.
2. Strain the liquid into a second bowl. Discard the nettles.
3. With a spoon or whisk, blend the olive oil and chamomile essential oil into the liquid.
4. Using a soft cloth, dab the mixture onto the affected area, then air dry.
5. Repeat 2 to 3 times daily while hives persist.

JOINT & MUSCLE PAIN

You don't have to be a pro athlete or gym rat to experience joint and muscle pain. In fact, the simple act of everyday living can lead to the minor injuries that lead to strain and discomfort. Time, rest, and simple home remedies can bring fast, effective relief. Try these alone or alongside other remedies and complementary therapies like massage or acupuncture. If your pain worsens or fails to improve, check in with your care provider.

Cayenne Salve

YIELD: 8 OUNCES
STORAGE: GLASS JAR OR TIN
TIME: 48 HOURS FOR BREWING

Cayenne offers deep, penetrating heat that quickly eases joint and muscle pain. Be careful to keep this formula away from your eyes and wash hands thoroughly after preparing (use fresh lemon juice in a pinch).

½ cup cayenne pepper
7 ounces organic olive oil
1 ounce beeswax, grated

1. In a jar, combine the cayenne pepper and olive oil.
2. Cap the jar tightly and put it in a warm place for 48 hours.
3. Pour the oil through a fine sieve into a double boiler.
4. Add the grated beeswax and stir gently over low heat until the wax melts.
5. Cool the blend for 2 minutes.
6. Pour it into a jar or tin and cool completely before capping tightly.
7. Using your fingers, apply a thin layer to the affected area.
8. Use 2 to 3 times daily to stop pain. Store in a cool, dark place.

Cooling Mint Compress

YIELD: 1 TREATMENT
STORAGE: NOT RECOMMENDED
TIME: 20 MINUTES

That refreshing zing that peppermint gives your senses is the same effect it has on your circulation, triggering an increase in blood flow that stops pain and swelling. After applying the compress, elevate the injured area to bring further relief.

2 cups cold water
2 cups ice
½ teaspoon organic olive oil
5 drops peppermint essential oil

1. In a large bowl, combine the water and ice.
2. In the palm of your hand, combine the olive oil and peppermint essential oil.
3. Rub the oils onto the affected area.
4. Soak a soft cloth in the ice water and wring out the excess moisture.
5. Apply the cloth to the affected area, covering the oils.
6. Relax for 20 minutes or so, refreshing the cloth with more cold water.
7. Repeat 2 to 3 times daily.

Arnica-Peppermint Liniment

YIELD: 1 PINT
STORAGE: DARK-COLORED GLASS BOTTLE OR JAR
TIME: 4 WEEKS

Soreness will retreat in the face of a quadruple threat from arnica, peppermint, cayenne, and goldenseal. Because this preparation takes several weeks to mature, it's best to make it before you need it. If you regularly suffer from joint or muscle soreness, or have some intensive physical activity lined up, don't delay in putting this together. The mixture lasts indefinitely when properly stored.

1 pint rubbing alcohol
4 tablespoons dried arnica flowers
4 tablespoons dried peppermint leaves
2 tablespoons goldenseal powder
1 tablespoon cayenne powder
1 teaspoon peppermint essential oil

1. In a 1-quart canning jar, combine the rubbing alcohol, arnica, peppermint leaves, goldenseal, and cayenne. Cap the jar tightly and shake well.
2. Place the jar in a warm area. Shake it once daily for a month.
3. When four weeks have passed, strain the liquid into a glass pitcher, discarding the herbs.
4. Add the peppermint essential oil and mix well.
5. Pour the finished liniment into a dark-colored glass bottle or jar (a sterilized wine bottle works well).
6. Apply to the affected area with a cotton pad and allow to air dry. Reapply as often as needed.

LARYNGITIS

Usually brought on by excess coughing due to a cold, bronchitis, or another illness, laryngitis typically lasts for three days to three weeks. Use these herbal remedies alongside other treatments, and let your doctor know if the problem lasts for more than three days in case an infection is to blame.

Cayenne-Myrrh Gargle

YIELD: 4 OUNCES
STORAGE: NOT RECOMMENDED
TIME: 5 MINUTES

Cayenne and myrrh combine with apple cider vinegar to bring relief while reducing bacteria. This gargle is good for sore throats, too.

2½ ounces warm water
1 ounce apple cider vinegar
1 tablespoon honey
1 teaspoon cayenne pepper
2 drops myrrh essential oil

1. In a glass, combine all the ingredients.
2. Stir well to blend.
3. Gargle with 1 mouthful of the solution at a time, spitting it out afterward.
4. Repeat until all of the solution is gone.
5. Rinse your mouth with water.
6. Use 2 to 3 times daily.

Goldenseal-Ginger Infusion

YIELD: 1 CUP
STORAGE: NOT RECOMMENDED
TIME: 15 MINUTES

Sore throats love this comforting mixture of spicy-sweet ingredients designed to soothe irritation and promote healing in minutes. With a generous dollop of honey, your taste buds won't be complaining either.

1 teaspoon peeled, grated fresh ginger root
1 teaspoon dried goldenseal
1 teaspoon lemon juice
1 tablespoon honey
1¼ cups water

1. In a small saucepan, combine all the ingredients. Bring to a boil.
2. Reduce the heat to medium-low and simmer for 10 minutes.
3. Strain into a mug, using the back of a spoon to press the liquid from the ginger and goldenseal before discarding them.
4. Drink 2 to 3 times daily when suffering from laryngitis.

Echinacea-Clove Throat Spray

YIELD: 1 TREATMENT
STORAGE: NOT RECOMMENDED
TIME: 5 MINUTES

Echinacea combats infection and inflammation, making it ideal for easing laryngitis symptoms. Fresh ginger root and clove essential oil combine to numb the pain and kill bacteria.

½ cup boiling water
1 tablespoon chopped dried echinacea root
1 teaspoon peeled, finely grated fresh ginger root
2 drops clove essential oil

1. In a cup, combine the water, dried echinacea root, and fresh grated ginger root.
2. Allow the mixture to cool completely.
3. Strain the liquid into a small glass pitcher and discard the herbs.
4. Transfer the liquid into a 4-ounce spray bottle.
5. Add the clove essential oil and shake well.
6. Spray into your mouth, aiming for the back of the throat.
7. Wait at least 10 minutes before eating or drinking. Use as often as needed.

NAUSEA/ MORNING SICKNESS

Whether you're battling morning sickness, motion sickness, or the kind of nausea that comes along with the flu, herbal remedies can often bring quick relief from your misery. Use these gentle but potent natural treatments alone or in combination with another to feel more like yourself again.

Ginger Smelling Salt

YIELD: 1 OUNCE
STORAGE: SMALL GLASS JAR
TIME: 2 MINUTES

The aroma of ginger essential oil is a powerful weapon in your arsenal against nausea. This smelling salt is a good choice for nausea associated with motion sickness and morning sickness, too.

1 ounce coarse sea salt
20 drops ginger essential oil

1. In a small glass jar, combine the sea salt with the ginger essential oil.
2. Shake well to blend.
3. Cap tightly.
4. Inhale deeply for 10 to 15 seconds when feeling nauseous.
5. Use as often as needed. When the fragrance starts to fade, refresh with additional essential oil.

Peppermint-Ginger Tea

YIELD: ABOUT 1 CUP
STORAGE: NOT RECOMMENDED
TIME: 15 MINUTES

Peppermint and ginger combine to help the digestive tract to relax, easing the muscle spasms that lead to feelings of nausea.

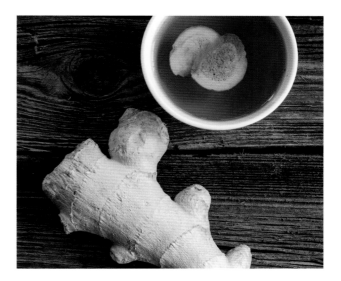

1 tablespoon crushed dried peppermint leaves
1 teaspoon peeled, grated fresh ginger root
1¼ cups boiling water
Honey or stevia (optional)

1. Put the peppermint leaves and ginger root in a tea ball or infuser. Place the tea ball in a mug of the boiling water.
2. Steep the herbs for 15 minutes.
3. Sweeten with honey or stevia, if desired, and drink the tea while relaxing. Enjoy as often as needed.

POISON IVY

No trek through the great outdoors seems to be complete without at least one unfortunate run-in with poison ivy, poison oak, or poison sumac, all of which cause itching, redness, and pain. These symptoms are caused by an irritant called urushiol, an oily resin that sticks to skin, clothing, gardening tools, and other items. See your doctor if your eyes or mucus membranes are affected, or if the rash seems to be spreading.

Peppermint Spray

YIELD: 4 OUNCES
STORAGE: GLASS BOTTLE WITH SPRAY TOP
TIME: 5 MINUTES

Peppermint essential oil cools burning and soothes itching quickly. Use this remedy immediately after bathing or showering.

4 ounces unflavored vodka
20 drops peppermint essential oil

1. In a glass bottle, combine the vodka and peppermint essential oil.
2. Cap tightly and shake well before each use.
3. Spray directly onto the affected area.
4. Let the area dry before dressing.
5. Repeat as often as needed.

Eucalyptus-Lavender Spray

YIELD: 4 OUNCES
STORAGE: GLASS BOTTLE WITH SPRAY TOP
TIME: 5 MINUTES

Get your cool on with this healing mix of eucalyptus, lavender, and witch hazel. One spray spritzes away itching and burning and leaves skin feeling calmer and more refreshed.

1 tablespoon eucalyptus essential oil
1 tablespoon lavender essential oil
3 ounces alcohol-free witch hazel extract

1. In a glass bottle, add the eucalyptus and lavender essential oils to the witch hazel extract.
2. Cap tightly and shake well before each use.
3. Spray directly onto the affected area.
4. Let the area dry before dressing.
5. Repeat as often as needed.

Peppermint-Kelp Bath

YIELD: 1 TREATMENT
STORAGE: NOT RECOMMENDED
TIME: 30 MINUTES

If you anticipate a run-in with poison ivy, keep the peppermint essential oil, dried kelp, and sea salt on hand so they're readily available when you need them. The sooner after exposure you use this treatment, the better it works.

10 drops peppermint essential oil
3 tablespoons dried kelp, wrapped in cheesecloth
3 tablespoons Dead Sea salt or Himalayan sea salt
½ cup baking soda

1. Run a cool bath and add all of the ingredients.
2. Submerge yourself in the tub and soak for at least 30 minutes.
3. Pat your body dry when finished. Apply Peppermint Spray (opposite), Eucalyptus-Lavender spray (left), or another leave-on poison ivy remedy.
4. Put on loose clothing made of a natural fiber such as cotton.
5. Enjoy this healing bath once or twice daily while suffering from poison ivy.

PMS

If you're reading this section, you probably know firsthand that headaches, mood swings, bloating, and fatigue are just some of the symptoms that accompany PMS. Triggered by hormonal changes associated with your monthly cycle, symptoms can start two weeks prior to your period and make you miserable for days on end once it starts. Next time you're suffering, seek relief using these simple herbal remedies, either alone or as a complement to others.

Black Cohosh–Raspberry Leaf Infusion

YIELD: 1 CUP
STORAGE: NOT RECOMMENDED
TIME: 10 MINUTES

Black cohosh and raspberry leaf combine to balance hormonal levels and relieve discomfort caused by tension and cramping.

1 tablespoon dried black cohosh
1 tablespoon crumbled dried raspberry leaf
1 tablespoon honey
1¼ cups water

1. In a small saucepan, add the black cohosh, raspberry leaf, and honey to the water. Bring to a boil.
2. Reduce the heat and simmer the mixture for 10 minutes.
3. Strain into a mug, using the back of a spoon to press the liquid from the herbs before discarding them.
4. Drink 2 to 3 cups daily while suffering from PMS symptoms.

Herbal PMS Bath Salt

YIELD: 4 CUPS
STORAGE: AIRTIGHT CONTAINER
TIME: 20 MINUTES

This essential oil blend will lift your mood and fight depression, while the warm bath water will help ease discomfort. Make this bath salt ahead of time for convenience.

4 cups Epsom salt
40 drops geranium essential oil
20 drops chamomile essential oil
12 drops clary sage essential oil
8 drops marjoram essential oil

1. In an airtight container, add all the ingredients. Stir well to combine.
2. Draw a warm bath.
3. Add 1 cup of the bath salt and let it dissolve.
4. Spend 15 to 20 minutes soaking. Breathe deeply while enjoying.
5. Repeat as often as you like.

All-Around PMS Massage Oil

YIELD: 1 TREATMENT
STORAGE: NOT RECOMMENDED
TIME: 10 MINUTES

Targeting both cramps and mood swings, this six-oil blend is a powerful way to address all of the symptoms of PMS. If you're missing an oil or two, don't worry. This remedy works best with all ingredients, but it will provide some relief even if one or two ingredients are left out.

1 ounce coconut oil, warmed to 90 degrees
2 drops chamomile essential oil
2 drops clary sage essential oil
2 drops geranium essential oil
2 drops ginger essential oil
2 drops lavender essential oil
2 drops marjoram essential oil

1. In a small dish, combine the warm coconut oil with all of the essential oils.
2. Using your fingertips, massage generously into the lower abdomen, hips, and lower back.
3. Allow the treatment to fully absorb.
4. Apply the massage oil once or twice daily while PMS symptoms persist. If you have time, enjoy a hot bath before applying it.

SINUSITIS

You're sneezing, blowing your nose, feeling congested. Must be a cold, right? Maybe, maybe not, but the symptoms are the same. When the delicate tissue that lines your sinuses becomes inflamed and swollen, mucus and air are trapped inside, leading to pain and pressure. Speed relief by using these herbal remedies along with conventional treatments. This condition can be a serious problem, so let your doctor know if symptoms persist for more than a week or so.

Eucalyptus Sinus Steam

YIELD: 1 TREATMENT
STORAGE: NOT RECOMMENDED
TIME: 20 MINUTES

Eucalyptus opens blocked sinuses quickly. The vapors from this treatment penetrate deeply, helping to kill harmful bacteria in the process.

4 cups boiling water
2 drops eucalyptus essential oil

1. In a shallow bowl, combine the boiling water and eucalyptus essential oil.
2. Place the bowl on a tabletop and sit comfortably in front of it.
3. Cover the bowl and your head with a large towel.
4. Breathe the vapors while relaxing and come out for air as needed. Keep tissues handy.
5. Use once or twice daily while recovering from sinusitis.

Herbal Shower Steam

YIELD: 1 TREATMENT
STORAGE: NOT RECOMMENDED
TIME: 15 MINUTES

The essential oils in this remedy combine to alleviate sinusitis symptoms while you're enjoying your daily shower. If you are missing one or two of them, use a little more of whichever oils you do have on hand.

2 drops eucalyptus essential oil
2 drops lavender essential oil
2 drops peppermint essential oil
2 drops rosemary essential oil

1. Drip the essential oils onto a washcloth.
2. Place the washcloth in the shower, positioning it opposite the drain.
3. Breathe deeply while enjoying a hot shower.
4. Enjoy this treatment once or twice daily while dealing with sinusitis symptoms.

Eucalyptus-Rosemary Smelling Salt

YIELD: 1 OUNCE
STORAGE: SMALL GLASS JAR
TIME: 5 MINUTES

Eucalyptus and rosemary work in concert to knock out stuffiness and other discomforts associated with sinusitis. This remedy is easy to take along so you can enjoy quick relief as needed.

1 ounce coarse sea salt
20 drops eucalyptus essential oil
20 drops rosemary essential oil

1. In a small glass jar, combine all of the ingredients.
2. Close the jar tightly and shake well to blend.
3. Remove the cap or lid and place your nose over the opening, inhaling deeply for 20 seconds.
4. Inhale this smelling salt as often as needed. If you notice that the aroma is beginning to fade after several uses, refresh the salt by adding another 10 to 20 drops of each essential oil.

♥ When you are over your illness and no longer need the smelling salts, transform them into bath salts. Add 10 drops of lavender essential oil and rinse the jar out into the bathtub while drawing a warm bath for yourself.

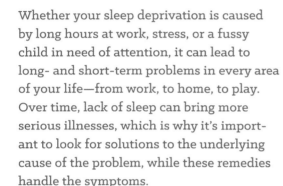

SLEEP DEPRIVATION

Whether your sleep deprivation is caused by long hours at work, stress, or a fussy child in need of attention, it can lead to long- and short-term problems in every area of your life—from work, to home, to play. Over time, lack of sleep can bring more serious illnesses, which is why it's important to look for solutions to the underlying cause of the problem, while these remedies handle the symptoms.

Chamomile–Valerian Infusion

YIELD: 1 CUP
STORAGE: NOT RECOMMENDED
TIME: 10 MINUTES

Chamomile and valerian combine to reduce the amount of time it takes you to fall asleep. Drink this infusion 30 minutes before bed.

1 tablespoon dried valerian
1 teaspoon dried chamomile flowers
1¼ cups water

1. In a small saucepan, add the valerian and chamomile flowers to the water. Bring to a boil.
2. Reduce the heat to medium-low and simmer the herbs for 10 minutes.
3. Drink 1 cup nightly as often as necessary.

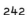 This infusion can be sedating. Do not use before driving or undertaking other tasks that require intense focus.

Hops Infusion

YIELD: 1 CUP
STORAGE: NOT RECOMMENDED
TIME: 15 MINUTES

Offering strong sedative properties, hops work as a natural sleep aid. Be sure to crush the hops well before adding them to the infusion.

1 tablespoon crushed hops
1 tablespoon honey
1 teaspoon lemon juice
1¼ cups water

1. In a small saucepan, add the hops, honey, and lemon juice to the water. Bring to a boil.
2. Reduce the heat to medium-low and simmer the mixture for 10 minutes.
3. Strain into a mug, using the back of a spoon to press the liquid from the hops before discarding them.
4. Drink 1 cup nightly for as many nights as necessary.

This infusion can be sedating. Do not use before driving or undertaking other tasks that require intense focus.

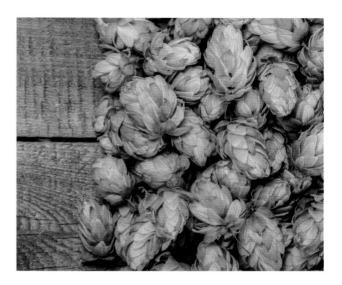

SORE THROAT

Sore throats can come from lifestyle habits, like public speaking, singing, or coaching. Or, they can be one of the first signs of ailments such as colds or strep throat. These soothing remedies knock out discomfort just as fast as an over-the-counter lozenge, sans the sugar and preservatives, regardless of the pain trigger. Use them alone to bring relief, or combine them with treatments for other symptoms as part of a complete natural healing plan for sickness.

Licorice Infusion with Slippery Elm

YIELD: 1 CUP
STORAGE: NOT RECOMMENDED
TIME: 15 MINUTES

Licorice and slippery elm powder combine with honey and lemon to coat your throat, bringing comfort quickly.

1 tablespoon chopped dried licorice root
2 teaspoons slippery elm powder
1 tablespoon honey
1 tablespoon lemon juice
1¼ cups water

1. In a small saucepan, combine all the ingredients.
2. Bring to a boil.
3. Reduce the heat to medium-low and allow the herbs to simmer for 10 minutes.
4. Strain into a mug, using the back of a spoon to press the liquid from the herbs before discarding them.
5. Drink 2 to 3 cups daily while recovering.

Ginger-Cayenne Gargle

YIELD: ABOUT 4 OUNCES
STORAGE: NOT RECOMMENDED
TIME: 5 MINUTES

Ginger and cayenne combine with lemon and honey to relieve your sore throat, bringing instant relief from the pain.

¼ cup warm water
1 tablespoon honey
2 tablespoons lemon juice
1 pinch cayenne pepper
1 pinch ground ginger

1. In a cup, combine all the ingredients, stirring to blend thoroughly.
2. Gargle with 1 tablespoon of the solution at a time, using the entire amount.
3. Repeat 2 to 3 times daily while recovering.

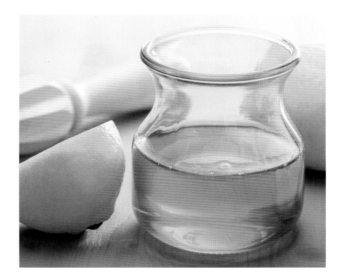

SPRAIN/STRAIN

Minor sprains and strains can easily happen any time you fall, twist a limb, or lift something a little too heavy for your muscles to handle. If pain and swelling are minor, these treatments, along with rest, elevation, and a cold pack, may be enough to heal the injury. Be sure to see your doctor if you don't see an improvement or if the pain gets worse.

Soothing Aloe Vera–Ginger Gel

YIELD: 8 OUNCES
STORAGE: PLASTIC SQUEEZE BOTTLE
TIME: 5 MINUTES

Think of the aloe vera in this treatment as a vehicle for delivering the warming, pain-relieving ingredients from the ginger deep into injured tissues. If you have no ginger essential oil on hand, use peppermint instead.

1 (8-ounce) bottle alcohol-free aloe vera gel
1 teaspoon ginger essential oil

1. In a large bowl, combine the aloe vera gel and ginger essential oil. With a whisk, stir well to blend.
2. Using a funnel, transfer the gel to a plastic squeeze bottle.
3. Apply a teaspoon of gel to the injured area. Massage gently.
4. Repeat 2 to 3 times daily. Refrigerate between uses.

Peppermint-Arnica Salve

YIELD: ABOUT 8 OUNCES
STORAGE: GLASS JAR OR TIN
TIME: 15 MINUTES

Peppermint and arnica combine to penetrate injured tissue, easing pain and swelling. Use ginger essential oil if you have no peppermint on hand.

3 ounces coconut oil
3 ounces organic olive oil
1 ounce beeswax, grated
1 teaspoon arnica essential oil
1 teaspoon peppermint essential oil

1. In a double boiler, combine the coconut oil, olive oil, and beeswax.
2. Stir gently over low heat until the beeswax melts completely.
3. Remove from the heat and cool for 2 minutes.
4. Add the arnica and peppermint essential oils.
5. Pour into a jar or tin and cool completely before capping tightly.
6. Apply a thin layer of salve to the injured area, massaging gently.
7. Use 2 to 3 times daily while recovering. Store in a cool, dark place between uses.

Quick Arnica-Sage Liniment

YIELD: 1 PINT
STORAGE: DARK-COLORED GLASS BOTTLE OR JAR
TIME: 5 MINUTES

Liniments made with fresh herbs take weeks to mature. This remedy is a quick one that can be used the same day it is mixed. The secret lies in the essential oils. Both arnica and sage penetrate deeply, delivering some relief from discomfort while encouraging damaged tissue to heal.

1 pint rubbing alcohol, vodka, or everclear
1 teaspoon arnica essential oil
1 teaspoon sage essential oil

1. In a glass bottle or jar with a tight-fitting lid, combine all of the ingredients.
2. Shake well before each use.
3. With a cotton pad or soft cloth, apply a thin layer of liniment to the affected area.
4. Allow the liniment to evaporate before dressing.
5. Apply 2 to 3 times daily while recuperating from a sprain or strain. Use it alone for minor injuries or alongside pain medication and other therapies.

TOOTHACHE

There are a number of issues that can cause teeth to hurt, some dental (say, tooth decay, abscessed teeth, damaged fillings, or infected gums) and others lifestyle (stress-related clenching, for instance). Both types can cause pain and swelling, and luckily, the pain can be treated with herbal remedies. Your dentist may offer additional treatments if your toothache is severe or lasts longer than two days. Earaches, fevers, and jaw pain are signs you should see a doctor, stat.

Clove Rinse

YIELD: ABOUT 8 OUNCES
STORAGE: GLASS BOTTLE OR JAR
TIME: 2 MINUTES

Cloves numb pain quickly, thanks to an anesthetic compound called eugenol. If you have no clove essential oil on hand, you can tuck a whole clove into your mouth and hold it next to the sore tooth.

8 ounces unflavored vodka
½ teaspoon clove essential oil

1. In a glass bottle or jar, combine the vodka and clove essential oil.
2. Shake well to blend before each use.
3. Rinse your mouth with 1 teaspoon of the solution, focusing on the sore tooth.
4. Spit the solution out after rinsing for 30 seconds to 1 minute.
5. Use once or twice daily while suffering from a toothache. Store in a cool, dark place.

Lavender-Chamomile Compress

YIELD: 1 TREATMENT
STORAGE: NOT RECOMMENDED
TIME: 20 MINUTES

Lavender and chamomile combine to ease pain and kill bacteria. You can use this treatment alone or alongside other remedies.

4 gauze squares
4 drops chamomile essential oil
3 drops lavender essential oil

1. Stack the gauze squares on top of one another.
2. Drip the essential oils onto the gauze.
3. Place the gauze onto the sore tooth.
4. Leave in place for 20 minutes.
5. Repeat twice daily.

Garlic Dental Compress

YIELD: 1 TREATMENT
STORAGE: NOT RECOMMENDED
TIME: 15 MINUTES

Fresh garlic contains allicin, a powerful antibiotic compound that also numbs pain. While packing fresh garlic onto a sore tooth might not sound like the best idea, this is a time-honored treatment that works wonders for pain while killing bacteria.

1 fresh clove garlic, peeled
1 pinch fine sea salt

1. With a sharp knife, carve a u-shaped channel lengthwise through the garlic clove. Try to make the channel roughly the same width as the tooth area you plan to use it on.
2. Sprinkle the salt into the channel and allow it to sit for 1 to 2 minutes, to draw out the garlic's juice.
3. Carefully position the garlic over the affected area and bite gently until you are certain the carved channel is in direct contact with the painful tooth.
4. Leave in place for at least 10 minutes, then discard. Do not eat or drink for at least 60 minutes.
5. Repeat this treatment as often as needed while waiting for your dental appointment.

WARTS

Warts are unsightly skin growths caused by a virus that infects the upper layer of skin. Be careful when treating them—you can inadvertently cause the virus to spread by touching a wart and then touching another body part, so take precautions to prevent this from happening. If these remedies fail to remove your warts, see your doctor for something stronger.

Garlic Compress

YIELD: 1 TREATMENT
STORAGE: NOT RECOMMENDED
TIME: OVERNIGHT

Garlic contains a powerful antiviral compound that can remove warts. This treatment must be repeated nightly over the course of 2 to 6 weeks.

1 clove garlic, peeled
Small bandage

1. Cut a small piece of garlic to fit the wart.
2. Cover the wart with the garlic.
3. Put the bandage in place. If needed, use athletic tape to make the bandage more secure.
4. Leave in place overnight.
5. Remove the bandage and the garlic in the morning. Speed the process by using this treatment during daytime hours as well.

Yarrow Compress

YIELD: 1 TREATMENT
STORAGE: NOT RECOMMENDED
TIME: OVERNIGHT

Fresh yarrow contains salicylic acid (the active ingredient that works like aspirin), which helps to remove warts naturally. This treatment must be repeated nightly over the course of 2 to 6 weeks for maximum results.

1 tablespoon fresh yarrow
Small bandage

1. Use a garlic press to obtain the juice from the yarrow.
2. With a cotton swab, apply the juice to the wart.
3. Cover the wart with the bandage.
4. Leave in place overnight.
5. Remove the bandage in the morning. Speed wart removal by using this treatment during daytime hours as well.

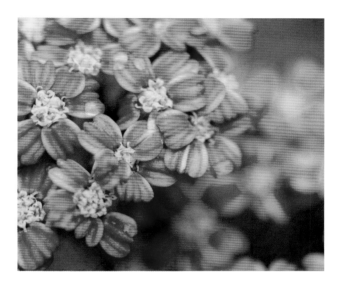

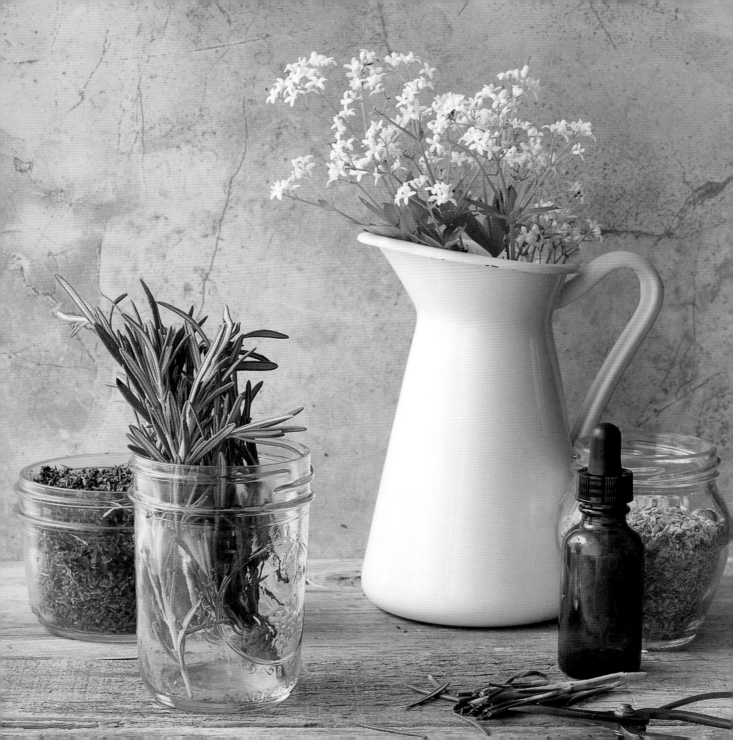

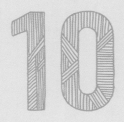

10

AROUND
THE HOUSE

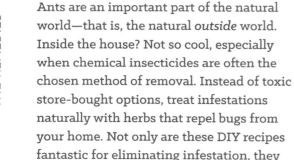

ANT INFESTATION

Ants are an important part of the natural world—that is, the natural *outside* world. Inside the house? Not so cool, especially when chemical insecticides are often the chosen method of removal. Instead of toxic store-bought options, treat infestations naturally with herbs that repel bugs from your home. Not only are these DIY recipes fantastic for eliminating infestation, they can also be used as fuss-free preventatives before insects make their way inside.

Garlic Ant Spray

YIELD: 1 GALLON
STORAGE: PLASTIC CONTAINER
TIME: 24 HOURS FOR BREWING

Garlic repels ants by confusing their sense of smell, which they rely on to create trails that lead from their nests to their food sources.

1 gallon boiling water
1 tablespoon liquid dish soap
6 full bulbs garlic, puréed

1. In a metal bucket, large glass or metal bowl, combine the water, dish soap, and garlic.
2. Cover the container and allow it to sit at room temperature for 24 hours.
3. Strain the liquid and transfer to a spray bottle for indoor use or a pump sprayer for outdoor use.
4. Apply liberally to areas where ants are a problem.
5. Store the unused portion in the refrigerator for up to 3 days. Freeze any extra.

❦ This spray is also effective against aphids and flea beetles. Like other topical solutions, this one needs to be reapplied after rain. Because garlic's natural scent dissipates, you may need to re-treat every few days until the ants move to a less hostile environment.

Peppermint Ant Repellent

YIELD: 1 TREATMENT
STORAGE: GLASS BOTTLE
TIME: 5 MINUTES

One of the easiest ways to get rid of ants indoors is to use peppermint essential oil straight out of the bottle it comes in. As an added benefit, this remedy leaves your home smelling minty fresh.

5 drops peppermint essential oil

1. Apply the peppermint essential oil to a cotton ball.
2. Wipe the area where ants have been seen.
3. Repeat with additional essential oil if treating a large area.

♥ This treatment keeps ants away for 3 to 4 days at a time, in most cases. Repeat it as necessary to prevent these pests from taking over.

Cayenne Ant Defense

YIELD: 1 TREATMENT
STORAGE: NOT RECOMMENDED
TIME: 5 MINUTES

This is a potent remedy that can cause discomfort to people (as well as ants) if it is inhaled or gets into your eyes. Handle cayenne powder cautiously and consider wearing rubber gloves. Diatomaceous earth, called for in this recipe, can be easily purchased online. It's best to wage ant warfare after dark, when most of the pesky insects are home in their nests. Plan for application before the sun goes down.

4 ounces cayenne powder
1 (4-pound) bag diatomaceous earth

1. In a bucket, combine both ingredients.
2. Using a scoop, apply a 1-inch-thick line of the mixture along areas where you have noticed ant activity.
3. If you know where anthills are located, surround the anthill with a heavy layer of diatomaceous earth and cayenne.
4. Leave in place for a few days, reapplying after rain.

♥ Diatomaceous earth is a food-grade, nontoxic powdery substance made from fossilized aquatic life. Nonetheless, it's best to keep curious children and pets away.

DISH DETERGENT

You don't need to pay a small fortune for expensive detergents full of chemicals. These natural solutions have what it takes to get dishes squeaky clean without the toxins. Made with simple ingredients that cut grease and remove stuck-on gunk, they smell fabulous and take just a few minutes to make.

Rosemary-Lavender Dishwashing Liquid

YIELD: ABOUT 20 OUNCES
STORAGE: PLASTIC SQUEEZE BOTTLE
TIME: 5 MINUTES

Rosemary and lavender essential oils give this natural dish soap a delightful fragrance, making a necessary chore more pleasant.

- **2 cups castile soap**
- **½ cup warm water**
- **3 drops rosemary essential oil**
- **2 drops lavender essential oil**

1. In a large bowl, combine all the ingredients. With a whisk, stir to blend.
2. Using a funnel, transfer the dish soap to a plastic squeeze bottle.
3. Shake well before each use.
4. Squeeze about a tablespoon of soap into a sink full of hot water.

❣ This dishwashing liquid is less sudsy than commercial brands. Do not use in dishwashers.

Clove Dishwasher Detergent

YIELD: 4 CUPS
STORAGE: SEALED JAR OR PLASTIC STORAGE CONTAINER
TIME: 5 MINUTES

Made with natural disinfectants and mild, natural abrasives, this fragrant dishwasher soap gets dishes clean without toxic chemicals. Use lavender, rosemary, or peppermint essential oil if you have no clove available.

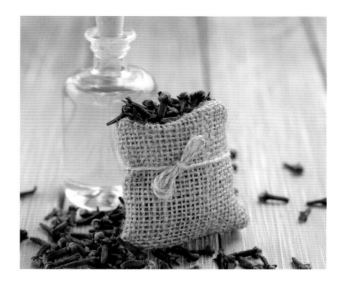

2 cups baking soda
20 drops clove essential oil
2 cups borax

1. In a large bowl, add ¼ cup of the baking soda.
2. Add the clove essential oil and mix well.
3. Add the rest of the baking soda and the borax, stirring to blend completely.
4. Using a funnel, transfer the powder to a storage container with a tight-fitting lid.
5. Fill your dishwasher's soap compartment and operate dishwasher normally.
6. Store in a cool, dark place.

♥ For best results, rinse heavily soiled dishes with water before putting them in the dishwasher. To eliminate spots on dishes, prevent odors, and reduce mineral buildup inside your dishwasher, fill the rinse compartment with white vinegar.

DISINFECTANT

Cleaners full of chemicals aren't necessarily the best defense against household dirt (especially when they add more toxins to your environment). These natural cleaning solutions work brilliantly on kitchens and bathroom surfaces, including countertops, sinks, and bathtubs. Their strong herbal ingredients cut grease and grime, kill germs, and leave your home sparkling clean. Best of all, they smell like a garden party.

Lemon-Eucalyptus Cleanser and Disinfectant

YIELD: 16 OUNCES
STORAGE: PLASTIC SPRAY BOTTLE
TIME: 5 MINUTES

This simple, inexpensive spray is tough on dirt while being easy on household surfaces. It kills germs naturally, leaving a fresh, sunny fragrance behind.

- **2 cups hot water**
- **2 teaspoons borax**
- **1 teaspoon washing soda**
- **8 drops lemon essential oil**
- **4 drops eucalyptus essential oil**

1. In a spray bottle, combine all the ingredients.
2. Cap tightly and shake well to mix.
3. Spray onto soiled surfaces and wipe with a rag or paper towel. For heavy soil, allow the cleanser to penetrate for 1 minute before wiping up.
4. Store in a cool, dry place between uses.

Rosemary-Lemon Soft Scrub

YIELD: 16 OUNCES
STORAGE: PLASTIC SQUEEZE BOTTLE
TIME: 5 MINUTES

Eliminate bathtub rings and other sticky, grimy messes with this nonabrasive scrub that leaves surfaces shining. Rosemary and lemon essential oils infuse the room with a refreshingly clean scent.

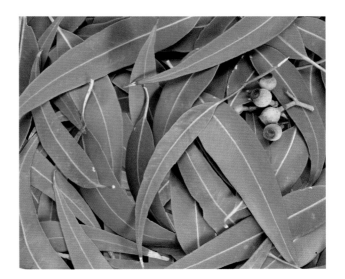

8 ounces borax
8 drops rosemary essential oil
8 drops lemon essential oil
8 ounces castile soap

1. In a large bowl, add the borax, rosemary essential oil, and lemon essential oil. Using a whisk, stir to blend.
2. Add the castile soap. Using a sturdy spoon, stir until a thick paste forms.
3. With a funnel, transfer the scrub to a plastic squeeze bottle.
4. Apply about a teaspoon of soft scrub to a sponge or brush and rub onto soiled areas.
5. Scrub vigorously to eliminate grime.
6. Store in a cool, dark place.

FLEAS

Warnings posted on conventional chemical-based flea repellents provide reason enough to look for natural, nontoxic solutions that are safe for you and your pets. Sure, you can use these indoor-outdoor remedies alone, but they're most effective when used together to address fleas outside as well as inside your home. Because natural treatments last for just a short time, vigilant reapplication is a must.

Lavender Flea Repellent

YIELD: ABOUT 4 OUNCES
STORAGE: GLASS BOTTLE
TIME: 5 MINUTES

These simple flea drops are safe for cats and dogs, and the lavender keeps fleas away. Be sure to avoid your pet's face when using, as essential oils can burn delicate eye tissue.

4 ounces olive oil
1 teaspoon lavender essential oil

1. In a glass bottle, combine the olive oil and the lavender essential oil.
2. Shake for 20 seconds to blend.
3. Pour a small amount of the solution onto your hand and rub it onto your pet's fur.
4. Store in a cool, dark place.

Use 5 to 6 drops for a cat or a small dog under 15 pounds, about ¼ teaspoon for a dog between 15 and 25 pounds, and ½ teaspoon for a dog weighing up to 40 pounds. For dogs over 40 pounds, apply 1 teaspoon at a time. Apply to outdoor pets daily. Others should be treated every 2 to 3 days.

Cedar–Witch Hazel Flea Spray

YIELD: 4 OUNCES
STORAGE: BOTTLE WITH A SPRAY TOP
TIME: 5 MINUTES

This natural flea repellent is ideal for your dog, and can be used on your shoes and trouser legs to help keep fleas and other bugs from hitching a ride while you're enjoying the outdoors.

4 ounces witch hazel extract
80 drops cedar essential oil

1. In a glass or plastic bottle with a spray top, combine the witch hazel and cedar essential oil.
2. Shake well before each use.
3. Spray onto your pet's fur.
4. Store in a cool, dark place.

For outdoor dogs, reapply daily. For dogs that spend most of their time indoors, reapply every 2 to 3 days. For cats, formulate a similar spray with lavender essential oil instead of cedar.

Lavender–Eucalyptus Flea Shampoo

YIELD: 2 CUPS
STORAGE: PLASTIC SQUEEZE BOTTLE
TIME: 5 MINUTES

Instead of bathing your pet with toxic chemicals, try this quick herbal flea shampoo made with old-fashioned hand dishwashing soap. While gentle on pets' sensitive skin, this thick, sudsy soap kills fleas by dissolving their exoskeletons.

2 cups dishwashing soap
1 teaspoon lavender essential oil
1 teaspoon eucalyptus essential oil

1. In a bowl, combine all of the ingredients and stir well to mix.
2. Transfer the soap to a plastic squeeze bottle. A clean shampoo bottle will do.
3. Wet your pet with warm water.
4. Scrub your pet with the shampoo, using enough to suds up the entire body. Be sure to apply in all of the places fleas like to hide—underarms, ears, beneath the tail, and between the toes.
5. Leave the suds on your pet for 5 minutes to be sure the fleas are killed.
6. Rinse thoroughly, towel dry, and give your pet a treat.

FURNITURE POLISH

Want to know a dirty little secret about store-bought cleansers? They're full of dangerous chemicals that aren't necessary to keep surfaces sparkling. Instead of spending top dollar for pricey furniture sprays and polishes, save money and enjoy greater peace of mind by whipping up your own solutions at home. These simple recipes contain ingredients you likely already have around the house, along with some essential oils that increase their efficiency while leaving an enjoyable fragrance behind.

Dusting Spray

YIELD: 8 OUNCES
STORAGE: PLASTIC SPRAY BOTTLE
TIME: 5 MINUTES

Treat wood furniture right with this fragrant dusting spray. With olive oil for shine and to protect wood from moisture, it contains essential oils to disinfect and impart fragrance.

¼ cup white vinegar
¾ cup olive oil
20 drops lavender essential oil
20 drops peppermint essential oil

1. In a plastic spray bottle, combine all the ingredients.
2. Shake well before each use.
3. Spray directly onto wood furniture or onto a soft cloth. Wipe to remove dust and grime.
4. For heavily soiled furniture, allow the polish to sit for 1 minute before wiping.
5. Store in a cool, dark place.

Lemon-Rosemary Furniture Polish

YIELD: 12 OUNCES
STORAGE: PLASTIC SPRAY BOTTLE
TIME: 5 MINUTES

If you love the fragrance of lemon furniture polish, you'll appreciate this all-natural version. It moisturizes wood while leaving a lovely shine and a pleasant lemon scent behind.

1 cup olive oil
½ cup lemon juice
20 drops lemon essential oil
5 drops rosemary essential oil

1. In a spray bottle, combine all the ingredients.
2. Shake well before each use.
3. Spray the cleaner onto a soft cloth. Wipe the furniture with the cloth, then use a second cloth to polish to a shine.
4. For heavily soiled furniture, allow the polish to sit for 1 minute before wiping.
5. Store in a cool, dark place.

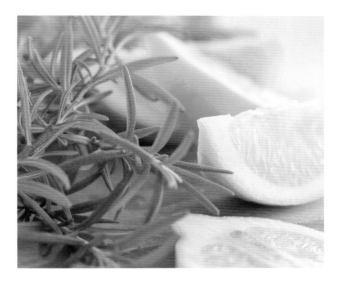

LAUNDRY

Ever notice that the all-natural laundry soaps available for purchase tend to cost more than their conventional counterparts? Creating your own laundry solutions at home gives you control of the ingredients, ensuring that the detergent you use is a good choice for your skin and the planet. These quick, easy recipes will help you save money while leaving clothes fresh and clean.

Herbal Laundry Soap

YIELD: ABOUT 5 CUPS
STORAGE: AIRTIGHT JAR OR PLASTIC CONTAINER
TIME: 10 MINUTES

This laundry detergent smells fantastic and gets clothes squeaky clean. Use a pure, unscented bar soap like Ivory, Fels-Naptha, or Dr. Bronner's for best results.

2 cups borax
2 cups washing soda
2 bars soap, grated
10 drops lavender essential oil
5 drops rosemary essential oil
5 drops peppermint essential oil

1. In a blender or food processor, combine all the ingredients.
2. Process on medium speed for 30 seconds.
3. Let the dust settle before removing the lid.
4. Transfer to a large glass jar or resealable plastic storage container.
5. Use 1 tablespoon of soap for a small load of laundry. Increase that amount to 2 or 3 tablespoons for larger loads or heavily soiled clothing.
6. Store in a cool, dry place.

Herbal Fabric Softener

YIELD: ½ GALLON
STORAGE: ORIGINAL VINEGAR BOTTLE
TIME: 5 MINUTES

You'll be amazed at how soft this fragrant fabric softener leaves your clothing. Experiment with different essential oil combinations if you like.

15 drops lavender essential oil
10 drops peppermint essential oil
10 drops rosemary essential oil
½ gallon white vinegar

1. Add the lavender, peppermint, and rosemary essential oils to the vinegar.
2. Shake well before each use.
3. Add ½ cup to the rinse cycle for average loads. If you have an HE washer, use ¼ cup.
4. Store in a cool, dark place.

Lemon Stain Remover

YIELD: 1 TREATMENT
STORAGE: NOT RECOMMENDED
TIME: 5 MINUTES

Stock your laundry room with lemon essential oil, baking soda, and hydrogen peroxide to work out tough stains as soon as they happen. The immediate chemical reaction between the ingredients in this remedy causes vigorous bubbling action that lifts the stain. The fresh reaction is what makes the mixture so effective, so storage is not recommended.

1 drop lemon essential oil
½ teaspoon water
½ teaspoon baking soda
1 teaspoon hydrogen peroxide 3%

1. Apply the lemon essential oil to a toothbrush designated for stain-removal use.
2. Moisten the stain with water, working from the outer edge toward the inside.
3. Sprinkle the baking soda onto the stain. Use more for a larger stain.
4. With the toothbrush, scrub the stain vigorously from outside to inside.
5. Rinse the toothbrush with water, then use it to apply the hydrogen peroxide to the stain, which should begin to bubble.
6. When the bubbling subsides, rinse the stain with water.
7. Repeat until the stain is gone. Most fresh stains are eliminated after 1 or 2 treatments.

MICE

Whether you perceive mice as cute or frightening, you don't want them in your home. Capable of causing extensive damage, harboring fleas, and spreading diseases, these troublesome little rodents belong outdoors. The good news is that you don't have to use chemicals or inhumane traps to keep them away. Because mice hate strong-smelling herbs, you can easily fend them off while making your home a more fragrant place to be.

Yarrow Mouse Repellent

YIELD: 6 CUPS
STORAGE: NOT RECOMMENDED
TIME: 5 MINUTES

The stronger the smell, the better an herb is at repelling mice. Yarrow is a very easy plant to grow. With its camphorous fragrance, it is one that mice hate.

6 cups fresh yarrow, chopped

1. Look inside your home for areas frequented by mice.
2. Sprinkle chopped yarrow along any trails and near potential entrances.
3. Repeat the process outdoors.
4. Reapply the yarrow every week or so to keep the mice from coming back. Dry more yarrow to use during the winter months, and apply it as often as needed to keep the scent strong.

♥ Yarrow can be toxic to cats, dogs, and horses. Keep out of their range.

Peppermint Mouse Bombs

YIELD: 30 MOUSE BOMBS
STORAGE: NOT RECOMMENDED
TIME: 10 MINUTES

Mice are sensitive creatures. They simply cannot stand the smell of peppermint and will stay away from areas where the odor is strong.

30 cotton balls
90 drops peppermint essential oil

1. Apply 3 drops of peppermint essential oil to each cotton ball.
2. Place the cotton balls around your home in areas where mice are active.

Periodically check to be sure that you can still smell the peppermint on the cotton balls. Once the scent is gone, mice will return. Walk around with your bottle of peppermint essential oil and refresh your cotton balls, or replace them with new ones.

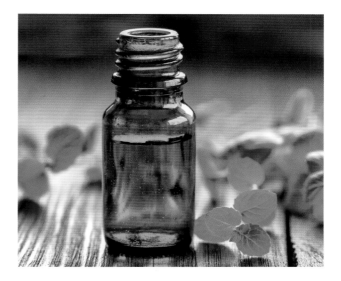

MOLD & MILDEW

Mold and mildew have a tendency to grow anywhere moisture and warmth are present, but they're no match for equally potent herbs. These fungi are often superficial and easy to remove from hard, non-porous surfaces, no harsh chemicals required. If you notice they keep returning despite your efforts to keep your home dry and well ventilated, invest in a professional assessment. Uncovering the source and addressing the problem early can help prevent costly repairs later.

Tea Tree Mildew Remover

YIELD: 3 OUNCES
STORAGE: NOT RECOMMENDED
TIME: 10 MINUTES

This potent mildew remover works on a variety of items, but may cause bleaching on dark-colored fabric. Start by testing it on a hidden area.

4 tablespoons salt
2 tablespoons lemon juice
12 drops tea tree essential oil

1. In a small bowl, mix together the salt, lemon juice, and tea tree essential oil.
2. Using a small, stiff brush, apply the cleaner to mildewed areas and scrub.
3. Leave the cleaner in place for 10 minutes.
4. Rinse with water.

If treating a fabric item, wash it in warm, soapy water. Rub the cleaner in, then place the item in full sunlight for 2 or 3 hours before rinsing. Repeat the process one more time if the stain persists.

Eucalyptus–Tea Tree Spray

YIELD: 8 OUNCES
STORAGE: SPRAY BOTTLE
TIME: 5 MINUTES

To prevent problematic mold and mildew in damp areas such as bathrooms, use this fresh-smelling antifungal spray during regular cleanups.

8 ounces white vinegar
12 drops eucalyptus essential oil
12 drops tea tree essential oil

1. In a spray bottle, combine the vinegar and the eucalyptus and tea tree essential oils.
2. Shake well before each use.
3. Spray onto soiled surfaces and wipe up with a cloth or paper towel. Store in a cool, dark place.

Lavender–Tea Tree Mold Scrub

YIELD: 1 TREATMENT
STORAGE: NOT RECOMMENDED
TIME: 5 MINUTES

If mold and mildew are causing stained grout or tile in the kitchen or bath, you'll find that this simple, inexpensive scrub is an effective, natural way to eliminate it. If the problem is severe, you may need to repeat the scrub and rinse cycle two to three times.

¼ cup baking soda
10 drops lavender essential oil
10 drops tea tree essential oil

1. In a cup or bowl, combine all of the ingredients, stirring with a whisk or fork.
2. Using a damp sponge, apply generously to the affected area.
3. Leave the mixture in place for 5 to 10 minutes.
4. Scrub the mixture with the sponge or a brush, using small circular motions, then rinse clean with water.
5. Use this solution any time you notice signs of mold or mildew returning. Apply the Tea Tree Mildew Remover (opposite) or Eucalyptus–Tea Tree Spray (left) to inhibit future growth.

MOTHS

Moths and other insects can damage clothing, furniture, and other fabric belongings. Still, you don't have to rely on your grandmother's methods for removal: mothballs. If you hate their distinctive smell and prefer not to use harmful chemicals in your home, you'll be happy to know that many plants protect themselves by emitting fragrances that naturally repel insects. Ironically, these same scents will seem pleasant to your nose and double as natural air fresheners.

Herbal Potpourri

YIELD: 1 CUP
STORAGE: PLACE IN AREAS AFFECTED BY MOTHS
TIME: 5 MINUTES

This herbal potpourri looks attractive in a bowl or jar, and can be sewn into sachets to hang in closets. Don't worry if you are missing one or two of the herbs. All are potent moth repellents.

- **1 tablespoon dried basil**
- **1 tablespoon dried bay leaves**
- **1 tablespoon dried rosemary**
- **1 tablespoon dried thyme**
- **4 tablespoons dried lavender flowers**
- **2 drops lavender essential oil**
- **2 drops rosemary essential oil**

1. In a bowl or jar, combine the basil, bay leaves, rosemary, thyme, and lavender flowers.
2. Sprinkle the lavender and rosemary essential oils on top and mix gently with your hands.
3. Stuff the potpourri into sachets or use it to fill a bowl, jar, or sugar shaker.
4. Place the potpourri in areas where moths are active.

❣ This blend loses its potency over time and needs to be replaced every 2 to 3 months.

Spicy Cedar Potpourri

YIELD: 4 CUPS
STORAGE: PLACE IN AREAS AFFECTED BY MOTHS
TIME: 5 MINUTES

Use this potpourri to make sachets to stash in closets or drawers. Fresh cedar chips can be found at stores that carry pet supplies.

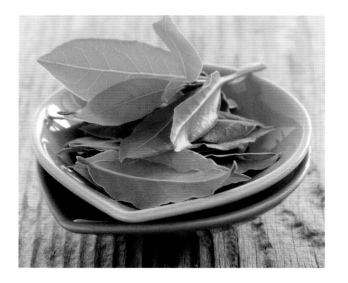

3 cups cedar chips
¼ cup whole cloves
¼ cup broken cinnamon sticks
¼ cup dried orange peel
8 drops cedar essential oil
8 drops clove essential oil
8 drops orange essential oil

1. In a large bowl, combine all the ingredients and mix with your hands or a large spoon.
2. Fill sachets, jars, bowls, or sugar shakers.
3. Place the potpourri in areas where moths are active.

♥ This blend loses its potency over time and needs to be replaced every 2 to 3 months.

PET ODOR

Pets make fantastic companions, but their odors don't. Keeping your home smelling Fido-free doesn't require harsh deodorizers that break the bank. Instead, test-drive these safe, natural deodorizers that emit a fragrance just as fresh as the chemical kind. Simple ingredients save cash and sidestep the worry that comes from sprinkling scented toxins all over carpets, rugs, and furniture.

Lavender–Tea Tree Carpet Powder

YIELD: 2 CUPS
STORAGE: SUGAR SHAKER
TIME: 5 MINUTES

This natural carpet powder absorbs pet odor and leaves a fresh, natural fragrance behind. Use it each time you vacuum to keep your home smelling its best.

2 cups baking soda
20 drops lavender essential oil
5 drops tea tree essential oil

1. In a large bowl, combine ¼ cup of the baking soda and the lavender and tea tree essential oils. Using a whisk or fork, mix well.
2. Add the remaining baking soda and stir well to combine.
3. Using a funnel, transfer the powder to the sugar shaker.
4. Sprinkle on your carpet 10 minutes before vacuuming. Store in a cool, dry place.

♥ For especially tough odors, leave the powder on the floor overnight and vacuum in the morning.

All-Purpose Lemon-Rosemary Disinfectant

YIELD: 8 OUNCES
STORAGE: BOTTLE WITH A SPRAY TOP
TIME: 5 MINUTES

Cleaning up wet pet stains is no picnic, but this natural disinfectant makes it easier. Use this cleanser on hard surfaces and carpet. Test it on a hidden area before use, as the lemon can lighten some dark colors.

- ½ cup rubbing alcohol
- ½ cup white vinegar
- 4 drops lemon essential oil
- 4 drops rosemary essential oil

1. In a bottle, combine all the ingredients.
2. Cap tightly and shake well.
3. When cleaning up wet pet stains, use a towel to blot up as much liquid as possible before application. Let the solution sit on the stain for 10 minutes, then wipe up. Work from the outer edge of the stain to its inside to keep it from spreading.
4. Spray the disinfectant over the stain. Let it sit for 10 minutes, then wipe up.

Rosemary Pet Stain Remover

YIELD: ABOUT 4 CUPS
STORAGE: 1-QUART GLASS JAR WITH TIGHT-FITTING LID
TIME: 20 MINUTES

Why pay high prices for special pet stain removers when you can make an equally effective homemade solution with simple ingredients? The rosemary essential oil will help deter pets from re-staining the same area, and this formula is gentle enough to use on most types of carpet and upholstery.

- 1 bar solid castile soap, chopped or grated
- 2½ cups boiling water
- ½ cup rubbing alcohol
- 1 teaspoon rosemary essential oil

1. In a glass quart jar, combine the castile soap and boiling water.
2. Stir until all the soap melts.
3. When the liquid has cooled, add the rubbing alcohol and rosemary essential oil.
4. Close the lid tightly and shake well. Shake again before each use.
5. To use, blot up as much of the stain as you can before beginning, then pour about a teaspoon of the stain remover onto a scrub brush.
6. Use the brush to scrub the stain, working your way from its outer edge to its center. Allow the solution to sit on the stain for 10 minutes before blotting up. Repeat until the stain is gone.

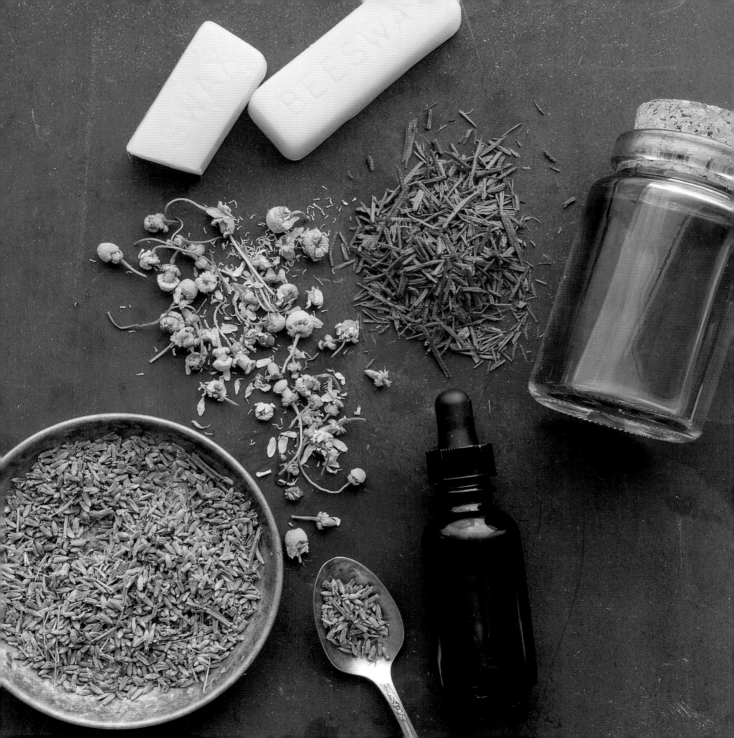

11

THE DAY AFTER

BREAKUP

Breakups stink so let's not pretend there are any easy cures for a broken heart. The best TLC often comes by indulging in life's healthier luxuries like ripe (organic) strawberries, a little dark chocolate, and plenty of one-on-one time with your best friends. In the meantime, soothe your mood by treating your body and mind to an aromatherapy bath with essential oils that help bring emotional healing.

Lavender–Bergamot Bath Salt

YIELD: 1 TREATMENT
STORAGE: NOT RECOMMENDED
TIME: 30 MINUTES

When blended, florally scented lavender and citrusy bergamot essential oils both miraculously chill you out and uplift your mood.

½ cup Epsom salt, sea salt, or Himalayan salt
1 tablespoon sunflower or olive oil
4 drops lavender essential oil
6 drops bergamot essential oil

1. In a small bowl, combine all the ingredients.
2. Draw a warm bath.
3. Add the bath salt and allow it to dissolve.
4. Spend 30 minutes soaking while breathing deeply.

DEATH OF A PET

When a pet passes on, the sense of grief and loss you feel can be overwhelming and disorienting. The grieving process takes time, but certain essential oils may make coping easier by relaxing tense muscles and calming your emotions. Some good ones to try include bergamot, chamomile, jasmine, frankincense, and lemon balm. Diffuse them or enjoy them in a warm bath, one or two essential oils at a time. Extra hugs are encouraged, too.

Soothing Bergamot-Chamomile Bath Oil

YIELD: 1 TREATMENT
STORAGE: NOT RECOMMENDED
TIME: 30 MINUTES

Bergamot and chamomile combine to relax body and mind. If you don't have time for a bath, combine the essential oils in this recipe with an ounce of sea salt and inhale deeply when you're experiencing emotional stress.

1 ounce olive or sunflower oil
3 drops bergamot essential oil
5 drops chamomile essential oil

1. Draw a warm bath.
2. Add all the ingredients and swirl with your hand.
3. Relax for 30 minutes while breathing deeply. Repeat as needed.

DRINKING BINGE

The morning after a drinking binge is never pretty. Instead of giving in to cheeseburger or taco cravings or countering a hangover with the hair of the dog, hydrate your body with good old H_2O and go back to sleep for a while. Eat something plain, starchy, and nutrient-dense—salads and smoothies are a good choice—to soothe your stomach and give your blood sugar a boost. Herbal remedies can help, too. Have some milk thistle to help your liver detox, and use herbal balms, like the recipe here, to soothe the pounding in your head.

Herbal Headache Balm

YIELD: 4 OUNCES
STORAGE: SMALL GLASS JAR OR TIN
TIME: 15 MINUTES

This magical pain reliever is the next best thing to having said no to that last drink. Make this calming balm ahead of time so you have it on hand when needed.

3 ounces organic olive oil
1 ounce grated beeswax
20 drops marjoram essential oil
20 drops peppermint essential oil
10 drops basil essential oil
10 drops chamomile essential oil
4 drops eucalyptus essential oil

1. In a double boiler, combine the olive oil and beeswax.
2. Over low heat, stir until the beeswax melts.
3. Remove from the heat and cool for 2 minutes.
4. Add the marjoram, peppermint, basil, chamomile, and eucalyptus essential oils.
5. Pour the balm into a small jar or tin.
6. Cool completely before capping tightly.
7. Apply a thin layer to the back of your neck and your temples and massage lightly.
8. Repeat as often as you like.

FENDER BENDER

Even a minor car accident can leave your body feeling sore and your mind in a fog. Not to mention the stress involved in dealing with other involved parties, insurance companies, tow-truck drivers, and police. Herbal teas are an excellent go-to when you need comfort, plus a medicinal kick to calm the nerves and relieve achy muscles.

Chamomile Chai Tea

YIELD: 1 CUP
STORAGE: NOT RECOMMENDED
TIME: 5 MINUTES

This comforting caffeine-free chai tea can easily be multiplied when the stress of the day calls for a double. For a livelier version, replace the chamomile and valerian with a plain black tea bag—but heads up, black tea contains caffeine.

- **1 tablespoon dried chamomile flowers**
- **1 tablespoon dried valerian**
- **¼ teaspoon ground cinnamon**
- **1 pinch ground ginger**
- **1 pinch freshly ground black pepper**
- **2 whole cloves, crushed**
- **1 cardamom pod, crushed**
- **1 tablespoon brown sugar**
- **1 cup cold water**
- **⅓ cup milk**

1. In a small saucepan, add the chamomile, valerian, cinnamon, ginger, black pepper, cloves, cardamom, and brown sugar to the water. Bring to a boil.
2. Reduce the heat to medium-low and simmer for 10 minutes.
3. Remove from the heat.
4. Strain into a mug, using the back of a spoon to press the liquid from the herbs and spices before discarding them.
5. Add the milk and stir before drinking.

HOME FROM THE HOLIDAYS

Holidays are supposed to be mini-vacations, but it's tough to get your life back on track after staying up too late, eating too much rich food, and engaging in the usual debates with family. Staying hydrated, eating right, and recommitting to an exercise habit will put you on the fast track to physical and emotional recovery. For extra support, incorporate herbs and essential oils into your health plan to help you bounce back from the stress of getting back to reality.

Energizing Licorice-Ginkgo Tonic

YIELD: 1 CUP
STORAGE: NOT RECOMMENDED
TIME: 15 MINUTES

With licorice and ginkgo, this tonic helps your body metabolize glucose better, plus it helps you recover from post-holiday fatigue.

1 teaspoon crushed dried ginkgo biloba
1 tablespoon chopped dried licorice root
1 tablespoon honey
1¼ cups water

1. In a small saucepan, add the ginkgo biloba, licorice root, and honey to the water. Bring to a boil.
2. Reduce the heat and steep for 10 minutes.
3. Strain into a mug, using the back of a spoon to press the liquid from the herbs before discarding them.
4. Drink 2 to 3 cups of tonic daily while getting back to your usual schedule.

INTERNATIONAL FLIGHT

After a long trip across time zones, you're likely to suffer from jet lag, complete with exhaustion, disturbed sleep, difficulty concentrating, and digestive issues. Herbal remedies work like magic to boost immunity and get sleep patterns back on track so you can avoid other issues that pop up after many days of planes, trains, and automobiles.

Goldenseal-Echinacea Immunity Infusion

YIELD: 1 CUP
STORAGE: NOT RECOMMENDED
TIME: 15 MINUTES

Goldenseal, echinacea, and ginger combine to boost immunity while helping your body recover from the exhaustion that often follows an international flight.

- **1 teaspoon dried goldenseal**
- **1 teaspoon dried echinacea**
- **2 teaspoons peeled, grated fresh ginger root**
- **1 tablespoon honey**
- **1¼ cups water**

1. In a small saucepan, add the goldenseal, echinacea, ginger, and honey to the water. Bring to a boil.
2. Reduce the heat to medium-low and simmer for 10 minutes.
3. Strain into a mug, using the back of a spoon to press the liquid from the herbs and grated ginger before discarding them.
4. Drink 1 or 2 cups each morning for 3 days.

❤ This treatment is also a good one for colds.

LAYOFF OR FIRING

It's normal to feel like you're on a roller coaster of tumultuous emotions after losing a job. Herbs aren't a magic elixir that can simply erase the anger, vulnerability, pain, or fear, but they can help you deal with the aftershock and reduce your stress. A clear head gives you the focus and empowerment you need to move forward in a productive, confident way.

Herbal Courage Balm

YIELD: 4 OUNCES
STORAGE: SMALL GLASS JAR OR TIN
TIME: 15 MINUTES

Lavender, chamomile, and ylang-ylang essential oils partner up with sandalwood to bring emotions back into balance so that you can gain the perspective needed to take positive steps. Bonus: Use this bravery booster whenever you need a shot of courage, like pre-interview or before speaking in public.

- 3 ounces olive oil
- 1 ounce grated beeswax
- 20 drops lavender essential oil
- 12 drops chamomile essential oil
- 8 drops sandalwood essential oil
- 8 drops ylang-ylang essential oil

1. In a double boiler, combine the olive oil and beeswax.
2. Stir gently until the beeswax melts completely.
3. Remove from the heat and cool for 2 minutes.
4. Add the lavender, chamomile, sandalwood, and ylang-ylang essential oils.
5. Pour into a small glass jar or tin.
6. Cool completely before capping tightly.
7. Apply the balm to hands, temples, or pulse points, breathing deeply for at least 20 seconds.
8. Use as often as you like.

MOVING HOUSE

There are few things more exciting—not to mention energy zapping, stress inducing, and muscle overloading—than move-in day. With your body and mind working overdrive, it's no wonder the day's activities leave you exhausted and depleted. Celebrate your next adventure with a few of your favorite treats, and then take a little well-earned time-out to break out the herbs and break in your new bathtub.

Arnica-Lavender Muscle Soak

YIELD: 4 CUPS
STORAGE: AIRTIGHT CONTAINER
TIME: 30 MINUTES

What's the next best thing to an Epsom salt bath? One that's spiked with arnica, lavender, and rosemary essential oils. It's just what the doctor ordered to relax tired muscles and promote mental relaxation.

4 cups Epsom salt
1 ounce calendula oil
½ teaspoon arnica essential oil
½ teaspoon lavender essential oil
10 drops rosemary essential oil

1. In an airtight container, combine all the ingredients.
2. With a spoon, stir well to blend.
3. Draw a warm bath.
4. Add 1 cup of bath salt and swish to dissolve.
5. Spend 30 minutes soaking while breathing deeply.

❦ Enjoy this bath any time you feel tired and sore. It's a fantastic one to use after workouts.

OVEREATING

The occasional food binge won't kill you, but it will make you feel sluggish almost immediately and for hours after the eating fest. Reenergize by drinking plenty of water or hot tea until your digestive system returns to normal. Chamomile and ginger are just some of the well-known herbs that can ease the symptoms of overeating. For a savory alternative, try this parsley infusion.

Parsley Infusion

YIELD: 1 CUP
STORAGE: NOT RECOMMENDED
TIME: 15 MINUTES

Fresh parsley can bring relief quickly by eliminating excess water weight. Try this infusion instead of nibbling on this flavorful herb all day.

3 tablespoons chopped fresh parsley
1¼ cups water

1. In a small saucepan, add the parsley to the water. Bring to a boil.
2. Reduce the heat to medium-low and simmer for 10 minutes.
3. Strain into a mug, using the back of a spoon to press the liquid from the parsley before discarding it.
4. Drink 1 cup up to 3 times daily while getting your digestive system back on track.

TV BINGE WATCH

Marathon viewing sessions are all the rage, but the downside of that sudden spate of sedentary behavior includes unpleasant side effects like fatigue or depression from lack of sunlight and social contact, a skipped shower or two, exhaustion from pulling all-nighters, and sluggishness from a three-day menu of pizza delivery. This quick herbal shower steam helps restore balance and brings you back to the real world.

Rosemary-Bergamot Shower Steam

YIELD: 1 TREATMENT
STORAGE: NOT RECOMMENDED
TIME: 5 MINUTES

This rejuvenating hit of rosemary, bergamot, basil, and peppermint will increase your energy level and motivate you to get things done. For extra staying power, hide the remote control.

6 drops bergamot essential oil
3 drops basil essential oil
3 drops peppermint essential oil
3 drops rosemary essential oil

1. Drip all the essential oils onto a washcloth.
2. Place the washcloth in the shower, away from the drain.
3. Spend 10 to 15 minutes showering while breathing in the invigorating aroma.
4. Use this aromatherapy blend any time you need to get up and get moving.

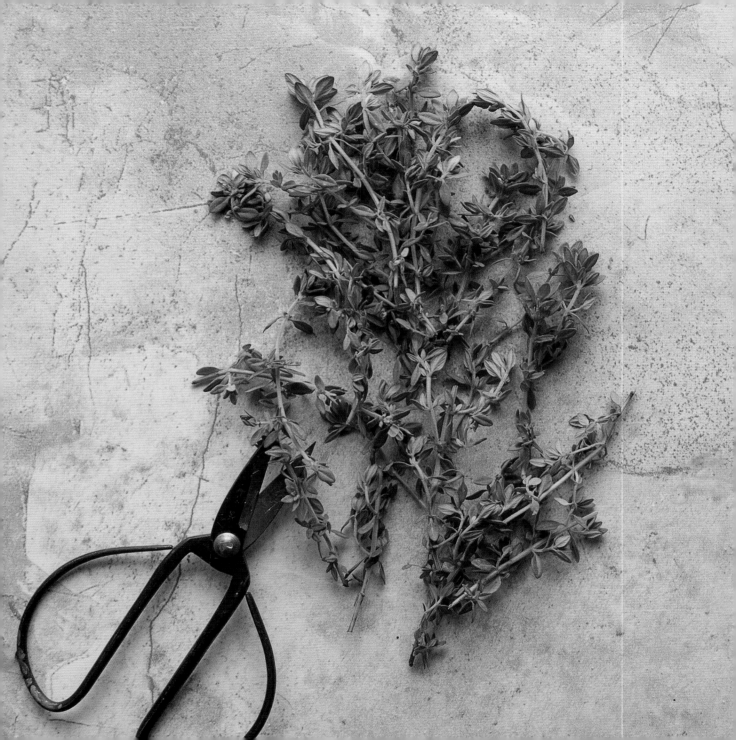

GLOSSARY

ADD (attention deficit disorder): A condition characterized by inattentiveness, often associated with, but not limited to, children.

ADHD (attention-deficit hyperactivity disorder): A chronic condition that begins in childhood and often extends into adulthood with symptoms of hyperactivity, impulsive behavior, and difficulty sustaining attention.

analgesic: A substance or compound that eases or stops pain.

antibacterial: A substance or compound that kills, reduces, or stops the growth of bacteria.

antifungal: A substance or compound that reduces or stops the growth of fungi.

antimicrobial: An agent that kills microorganisms or inhibits their growth.

antioxidants: Molecules found in plants, herbs, and food, like vitamins, that remove free radicals and other harmful oxidizing agents from your body.

antiseptic: A substance or compound that eases or stops the growth of infections.

antispasmodic: A substance or compound that stops spasms.

antiviral: A substance or compound that eases or stops the proliferation of viruses.

aromatherapy: A type of herbal medicine that uses essential oils and other therapeutic aromas to improve physical, mental, and emotional wellbeing.

astringent: A substance or compound that causes a constriction or contraction. Some herbs have an astringent effect on the pores of the skin.

Ayurveda: In Sanskrit, this term means "life knowledge." As a practice, it is a traditional Hindu system of alternative medicine.

botanical: A preparation made from part of a plant, as from roots, leaves, bark, or berries.

carotenoids: A class of naturally occurring pigments synthesized by algae, plants, and photosynthetic bacteria.

carrier oil: An oil that is used to dilute essential oils before they are applied to the skin.

compress: A piece of cloth that is soaked in the herbs and then applied to a particular part of the body.

corticosteroids: A class of chemicals that are produced in the adrenal cortex of vertebrates and tend to affect responses to stress and threats to the immune system and play a role in inflammation regulation.

decoction: A tea made by boiling the parts of a plant, like bark, roots, stems, and other woodsy components, in water to be used therapeutically. *See also* **infusion**.

diaphoretic: Pertaining to perspiration.

essential oil: Nutrient-dense oils extracted from parts of a plant, like stems, leaves, flowers, and fruits, which give off a specific healing aroma.

ethanol: Another name for alcohol. Often used to make tinctures.

exfoliant: An agent designed to slough off dead, dry cells from the skin.

expectorant: A substance or compound that expels mucous.

extract: A solution that contains the highly concentrated active ingredient of a substance.

flavonoids: Plant pigments that contain numerous antioxidants.

ginkgo biloba: A tree whose leaves improve blood flow to the brain and work as an antioxidant.

Hippocrates: An ancient Greek physician considered to be the father of Western medicine.

infusion: A tea made by pouring boiling water over delicate parts of the plant, like fruits, leaves, dried flowers, or berries, so the liquid steeps and the nutrients are imparted into the tea. *See also* **decoction**.

mask: A skin treatment used for detoxing, deep cleaning, and purifying skin head to toe.

mucilage: The thick, sticky substance inside plants that facilitates food and water storage and seed germination, plus houses many nutrients; it can be used in preparations.

naturopath: A licensed practitioner of therapy that relies on natural remedies to treat illness.

nutrient: A substance that provides nourishment and is necessary for growth and sustaining life.

pH level: A chemical scale from 0 to 14 that determines the amounts of acidity and alkalinity (pH greater than 7) of a substance.

poultice: A moist blend of organic materials designed to be placed on a piece of cloth and then applied to wounds and inflammation to stop pain, swelling, and soreness.

prebiotic: A nondigestible ingredient of food that promotes the growth of beneficial microorganisms in the intestines.

probiotic: A substance that promotes the growth of beneficial microorganisms.

rosacea: A skin condition characterized by facial redness, dilated blood vessels, bumps, and pustules.

salve: An ointment designed to heal, protect, or soothe the skin.

serum: A concentrated product used in cosmetology that contains geranium as a common ingredient.

tannin: A constituent found in plants that can be used for skin care as well as other treatments.

TCM (Traditional Chinese Medicine): An ancient medical practice that incorporates forms of herbal medicine, acupuncture, massage, exercise, and dietary therapy.

tincture: An herbal medicine created by combining plants with a solvent such as alcohol, vinegar, or glycerine. When applied topically and not orally, it is known as a **liniment**.

UVA (ultraviolet A)/UVB (ultraviolet B): Two types of harmful rays that come from sunlight. Raspberry provides protection from these effects.

HERBAL BEAUTY CARE KIT

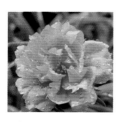 The recipes in this book offer plenty of room for creativity. The proportions suggested can be changed slightly to suit your taste, particularly when it comes to adding essential oils for aromatherapy. You can also add more or less liquid oil or beeswax to salves and balms to make them more fluid or thicker, and you can easily substitute oils and other ingredients for one another. Check out these additional ingredients to customize your DIY beauty kit.

Clays: Try bentonite clay in masks and poultices. It helps to absorb toxins and hold herbal remedies together. Green clay, red clay, and white or kaolin clay can be used as well. You can buy clays online and at some health food stores.

Cocoa Butter: If you're looking for a very rich, thick oil to use in place of coconut oil, cocoa butter can be a good choice. Use it sparingly on oily skin. Many drugstores carry cocoa butter.

Glycerin: This vegetable-derived additive draws moisture from the air to the skin. Use it to make lightweight lotions and creams. You can buy glycerin online and at specialty stores that carry supplies for making soap.

Hydrosols: Also known as flower water, hydrosols are a natural byproduct of the essential oil manufacturing process and are less expensive (and potent) than essential oils themselves. Use fragrances like chamomile, lavender, and rose to add unadulterated fragrances to your beauty products. Find them online and at stores that carry soap-making supplies.

Lanolin: A natural byproduct of wool, lanolin is a thick, waxy moisturizer. Look for it online.

Shampoo Base: This is an alternative to castile soap. Use it for making bubble bath, body wash, and of course shampoo. Look for it online and at health food stores.

MENTAL WELLNESS CARE KIT

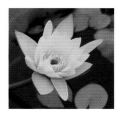 Using herbs for your mental well-being can involve making teas, tinctures, infusions, balms, bath salt, and much more. Make the process of total self-care a little easier by using some of the following tools.

Bath Pillow: Use an inflatable bath pillow to enjoy complete relaxation while taking herbal baths to ease stress and anxiety. They are easy to find at drugstores and department stores.

Essential Oil Diffusers and Pendants: With a diffuser, you can enjoy aromatherapy at home or at the office. Use an aromatherapy pendant to treat yourself to a constant stream of uplifting, soothing, or relaxing fragrance.

Meditation: There's no need to change who you are or spend a lot of money on a meditation coach. You can easily access guided meditations online, often for free. Use this tool to help bring your mind to the desired state quickly and easily.

Music: Soft music helps the mind relax, while songs with rhythmic beats promote an energetic feeling. Soothing music or the sounds of nature can help mask irritating noise and help you relax or sleep. Incorporate music into your herbal treatments to help foster the desired mood.

Tea Ball: Also known as a tea infuser, a tea ball is a small reusable strainer that holds dried herbs inside your cup or teapot, allowing the water to penetrate while making the brewing process a little bit tidier. Kitchen stores, department stores, and online retailers carry a variety of these tools.

RESOURCES

For more information, check out these retailers and helpful books.

Retailers

Annmarie Gianni Skincare

annmariegianni.com

Skincare and home products using natural, organic, and wild-crafted ingredients

Aura Cacia

auracacia.com

Essential oils and essential oil products

Banyan Botanicals

banyanbotanicals.com

Ayurvedic herbs in a variety of preparations

Dragon Herbs

dragonherbs.com

Herbs, tinctures, and teas

Horizon Herbs

horizonherbs.com

Seeds, culinary and medicinal herbs, plants, and trees

Jing Herbs

jingherbs.com

Medicinal herbs, teas, and tonics

Khushi Spa Products

khushispa.com

All-natural, organic spa and home products made with essential oils and herbs

Moroccan Elixir

moroccanelixir.com

Argan oil infused with organic essential oils for face, body, and hair

Mountain Rose Herbs

mountainroseherbs.com

Essential oils, aromatherapy, home, bath and body, containers, herbs, and more

National Institutes of Health

nih.gov

Medical research on herbal medicine

Rocky Mountain Oils

rockymountainoils.com

Organic essential oils

Seeds of Change

seedsofchange.com
Herbs, seeds, flowers, and supplies

Wei of Chocolate

weiofchocolate.com
Source for organic chocolate infused with
essential oils and herbs

Books

Bruton-Seal, Julie and Matthew Seal. *Backyard Medicine: Harvest and Make Your Own Herbal Remedies*. New York: Skyhorse Publishing, 2009.

Essential Oils Natural Remedies: The Complete A–Z Reference of Essential Oils for Health and Healing. Berkeley, CA: Althea Press, 2015.

Gladstar, Rosemary. *Rosemary Gladstar's Medicinal Herbs: A Beginner's Guide: 33 Healing Herbs to Know, Grow, and Use*. North Adams, MA: Storey Publishing, 2012.

Kastner, Mark and Hugh Burrows. *Alternative Healing: The Complete A–Z Guide to More Than 150 Alternative Therapies*. New York: Henry Holt and Company, 1996.

Lininger, Shulyer, ed. *The Natural Pharmacy*. New York: Harmony Books, 1998.

Tourles, Stephanie L. *Organic Body Care Recipes: 175 Homemade Herbal Formulas for Glowing Skin & Vibrant Self*. North Adams, MA: Storey Publishing, 2007.

Wardwell, Joyce A. *The Herbal Home Remedy Book: Simple Recipes for Tinctures, Teas, Salves, Tonics, and Syrups*. North Adams, MA: Storey Publishing, 1998.

Worwood, Valerie Ann. *The Complete Book of Aromatherapy and Essential Oils: Over 600 Natural, Non-Toxic & Fragrant Recipes to Create Health, Beauty, and a Safe Home Environment*. Novato, CA: New World Library, 1991.

REFERENCES

Akhondzadeh, S., H. R. Naghavi, M. Vazirian, A. Shayeganpour, et al. "Passionflower in the treatment of generalized anxiety: a pilot double-blind randomized controlled trial with oxazepam." *J Clin Pharm Ther.* 26, no. 5 (2001 Oct): 363–7. Accessed April 12, 2015. www.ncbi.nlm.nih.gov /pubmed/11679026.

American Cancer Society. "Ellagic Acid." Accessed April 13, 2015. www.cancer.org /treatment/treatmentsandsideeffects /complementaryandalternativemedicine /dietandnutrition/ellagic-acid.

Ashpari, Zohra. "The Calming Effects of Passionflower." *Healthline.* October 10, 2014. Accessed April 12, 2015. www.healthline .com/health/anxiety/calming-effects-of -passionflower.

Cassels, Caroline. "Active Compound in Rosemary May Be Neuroprotective." *Medscape Multispecialty.* November 15, 2007. Accessed April 13, 2015. www.medscape.com/viewarticle /565986.

Francis, Gabrielle, and Stacy Baker Masand. *The Rockstar Remedy: A Rock & Roll Doctor's Prescription for Living a Long, Healthy Life.* New York: Harper Wave, 2014.

Gladstar, Rosemary. *Rosemary Gladstar's Medicinal Herbs: A Beginner's Guide.* North Adams, MA: Storey Publishing, 2012.

Kastner, Mark and Hugh Burrows. *Alternative Healing: The Complete A–Z Guide to More Than 150 Alternative Therapies.* New York: Henry Holt and Company, 1996.

Li, Dandan, Jin M. Kim, Zhengyu Jin, Jie Zhou. "Prebiotic effectiveness of inulin extracted from edible burdock." *Anaerobe* 14, no. 1 (February 2008): 29–34.

Movafegh, A., R. Alizadeh, F. Hajimohamadi, F. Esfehani, M. Nejatfar. "Preoperative oral Passiflora incarnata reduces anxiety in ambulatory surgery patients: a double-blind, placebo-controlled study." *Anesth Analg.* 106, no. 6 (June 2008): 1728-32. doi:10.1213/ane .0b013e318172c3f9:1728-32.

Ohio State University, Wexner Medical Center. "Integrative Medicine: Our Director." Accessed April 9, 2015. wexnermedical.osu.edu /patient-care/healthcare-services/integrative -complementary-medicine/our-director.

Rabbani G.H., T. Butler, J. Knight, S. C. Sanyal, K. Alam K. "Randomized controlled trial of berberine sulfate therapy for diarrhea due to enterotoxigenic Escherichia coli and Vibrio cholera." *The Journal of Infectious Diseases* 155, no. 5 (May 1987): 979–84. doi:10.1093/infdis /155.5.979. PMID 3549923.

Salmalian, Hajar, Roshanak Saghebi, Ali Akbar Moghadamnia, Ali Bijani, et al. "Comparative effect of thymus vulgaris and ibuprofen on primary dysmenorrhea: A triple-blind clinical study." *Caspian Journal of Internal Medicine* 5, no. 2 (2014 Spring): 82–88. Accessed April 9, 2015. www.ncbi.nlm.nih.gov/pmc/articles /PMC3992233.

Srivastava, Janmejai K., Eswar Shankar, and Sanjay Gupta. "Chamomile: A herbal medicine of the past with bright future." *Molecular Medicine Reports* 3, no. 6 (2010 Nov 1): 895–901. Accessed February 25, 2015. www.ncbi.nlm.nih.gov/pmc/articles /PMC2995283.

Turker, A. U., and N. D. Camper. "Biological activity of common mullein, a medicinal plant." *Journal of Ethnopharmacol* 82, no. 2–3 (October 2002): 117–25. Accessed April 12, 2015. www .ncbi.nlm.nih.gov/pubmed/12241986.

Tveiten, D. and S. Bruset. "Effect of Arnica D30 in marathon runners. Pooled results from two double-blind placebo controlled studies." *Homeopathy* 92, no. 4 (October 2003): 187–9.

UCLA Health. "Mining Ancient Chinese Herbs for Cutting-Edge Therapies by Dr. Yung Chi Tommy Cheng, Yale University." Accessed April 9, 2015. exploreim.ucla.edu/video /mining-ancient-chinese-herbs-for-cutting -edge-therapies-by-dr-yung-chi-tommy -cheng-yale-university.

University of Maryland Medical Center. "Herbal Medicine." Accessed March 20, 2015. umm.edu/health/medical/altmed/treatment /herbal-medicine.

Wand, Shirley S. "Chinese Medicine Goes Under the Microscope." *Wall Street Journal.* April 2, 2012. www.wsj.com/articles/SB10001424052702 304177104577313821796467932.

OILS INDEX

REMEDIES INDEX

INDEX